健康人文英语

主　编　唐红梅　薛文隽
副主编　陆懿媛　沈　军

上海交通大学出版社
SHANGHAI JIAO TONG UNIVERSITY PRESS

内容提要

本教材内容兼具科学性和人文性，共包括十五个单元，分别对应十五个健康人文主题，围绕知识导向与价值认同、技能发展与思维塑造、家国情怀与融通中外等教育目标展开。每单元围绕单元主题，从健康人文视角全新切入，引用时代金句、中华文化，在语境中解读健康人文元素，通过阅读、翻译和思辨，在提升语言自信的同时，领悟中国智慧，讲好中国故事，传播中国声音。

图书在版编目（CIP）数据

健康人文英语 / 唐红梅,薛文隽主编. —上海：
上海交通大学出版社,2023.8（2024.8重印）
ISBN 978-7-313-28967-4

Ⅰ.①健…　Ⅱ.①唐…　②薛…　Ⅲ.① 医学—人文科
学—英语　Ⅳ.①R-05

中国国家版本馆CIP数据核字（2023）第116255号

健康人文英语

JIANKANG RENWEN YINGYU

主　　编：唐红梅　薛文隽
出版发行：上海交通大学出版社　　　　　　　　地　　址：上海市番禺路951号
邮政编码：200030　　　　　　　　　　　　　　电　　话：021-64071208
印　　制：常熟市文化印刷有限公司　　　　　　经　　销：全国新华书店
开　　本：787mm×1092mm　1/16　　　　　　印　　张：10.5
字　　数：170千字
版　　次：2023年8月第1版　　　　　　　　　　印　　次：2024年8月第3次印刷
书　　号：ISBN 978-7-313-28967-4
定　　价：49.80元

前　言

　　大学英语课程在通识教育中应具有人文性和工具性双重特征。我们以医学技术应用型人才培养为目标，策划、编写《健康人文英语》，供教师、学生和其他英语学习者使用。

　　大学英语人才培养工作旨在提升学生英语综合应用和跨文化交际能力的同时，培养学生的思辨能力，增强学生的文化自信。医学院校还应注重加强医者仁心教育，提升综合素质和人文修养，促进学科知识、语言能力和职业素养同步提升，培养有灵魂、有才干、有远见、有温度的学科人才。编撰本教材的初衷正是立足人文教育和学科建设，将知识传授、能力培养、价值引领有机结合，可作为广大院校师生选修教材。

　　本教材策划侧重实用性。在设计方面，注重通识教育与人文教育协调发展，对大学英语、学术英语等教材再开发，针对教材各单元主题摘编相关素材，深度挖掘人文元素；在选材上强调新颖有趣，贴近生活，引导深入思考，启发人生智慧。基于教材运用，整合资源，帮助使用者实现学用一体，具有良好的推广价值，助力彰显育人成效，推进新时期人才培养新局面。

　　本教材语言注重文学性。通过词语转译、词义引申，力求"信、达、雅"。选用优秀中华思想文化术语，例如，"贤哉，回也！一箪食，一瓢饮，在陋巷，人不堪其忧，回也不改其乐。贤哉，回也！""夫君子之行，静以修身，俭以养德，非淡泊无以明志，非宁静无以致远""凡大医治病，必当安神定志，无欲无求，先发大慈恻隐之心，誓愿普救含灵之苦"。书中语言积极向上，体现正能量，时事性强，在学习英语的同时又能感知汉语之美，美在形体，亦美在风骨，帮助我们从语言自信到文化自信，从健全人格到全面发展，促进科学和人文精神的结合，并将健康人文教育贯穿于学校教育、医务人员培训与继续教育阶段全过程。

本教材每单元由单元导入、主题摘编、育人金句、词汇宝典、应用提升、拓展阅读六部分组成。第一单元"爱国情怀"讲述爱国人士的感人故事，赓续红色基因；第二单元"美德雅颂"围绕中华传统美德，品读历史典籍，体会中华文化；第三单元"价值引领"强化社会主义核心价值观，学方法、得睿智，铸就科学世界观；第四单元"坚守信念"诠释奋斗使命，不忘初心，坚定信仰，谱写新篇章；第五单元"审美趣尚"根据新时代美育要求，感悟美学内涵，弘扬健康审美风尚；第六单元"艺术至上"着力寻求健康人文与艺术形式合理契合的要素，增强中华艺术认同感和获得感，发现艺术力量；第七单元"笃学之美"歌颂笃学敦行，修德精术，领略中华文化的独特魅力；第八单元"人文关怀"秉持学科及人文双螺旋发展，共情移情娓娓道来，致力健康中国；第九单元"求真探索"强调实践是检验真理的唯一标准，树立开拓精神，坚守科学真理；第十单元"大医精诚"呈现医学家仁心厚德、生命至上的楷模事迹，内化医者初心，接力济世强国；第十一单元"生态文明"阐释人与自然的关系，读懂美丽中国；第十二单元"绿色和谐"立足可持续发展、粮食安全与环保责任，理解和谐自然，保卫绿色家园；第十三单元"创新意识"介绍前沿科技发展，守正创新，点燃科技梦想；第十四单元"多元文化"旨在提高学生跨文化交际能力，恪守跨文化思维和意识，提升全球治理能力；第十五单元"全球视野"加强国际传播能力建设，拓宽全球视野，彰显世界胸怀。

本教材选入了不少名人名言，在收集时都已核对原文；在介绍其出处时考虑到教材并非专著，读者对象是学生，因此出处都尽可能简洁。

本教材在编写过程中得到了专家和同行的大力支持，他们不仅提供了精准专业的指导，还提供了及时高效的技术支持，在全书的撰写过程中付出大量心血，在此一并深表谢意。

由于编者水平有限，不妥之处，望使用者不吝赐教，以便进一步完善，不胜感激，联系方式：luyy@sumhs.edu.cn。

唐红梅

2023 年 8 月

Contents

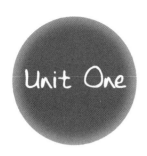

Unit One

Patriotism

Zhang Guimei, the principal of Huaping High School for Girls, based in Lijiang city, Yunnan province, has been granted the title "Role Model of the Times" in recognition of her dedication to the education for girls from poor families.

The school, which was founded by Zhang in 2008, was the first high school in the country to provide free education to girls who would otherwise have been unable to continue their studies after completing their nine years of compulsory education.

Anybody who knows Zhang's own conditions will be more deeply moved by her. She has no personal property, and has been living in the student dormitory since its founding. She has spent most of her salary and the bonuses she received on her students. And, despite having serious health problems, for 12 years she has always taken morning classes together with the students. She has also racked up 110,000 kilometers visiting her students' families over the years. Besides her work with the school, she also has a part-time job as head of the local orphanage, caring for more than 130 orphans.

Thanks to her efforts, about 40 percent of the school's graduates are enrolled in key universities. More than 1,800 girls from poor families have entered universities via her education.

Zhang deserves her honorary title. By helping the girls get higher education, she has actually helped them change their destinies, and their descendants in the future will enjoy more opportunities as a result. Influenced by her, many of her students have chosen to teach in poor areas, while some even went back to teach in her high school.

Now, with Zhang having got the honorary title, education for girls from poor regions will receive more attention, which hopefully brings more resources and assistance.

What she has done will be long remembered and encourage more to follow her example.

Questions:

1. Who is Zhang Guimei and what has she been doing since 2008?
2. Do you think Zhang Guimei's students who have chosen to teach in poor areas after graduating from university did the right thing? Why?
3. Do you have the courage to do something like what Zhang Guimei has been doing?

Part II Reading Task

● When I first came here, people were surprised to see a foreigner; it was something new, exotic. Today, Chinese people are going around the world, they are shoppers around the world, they are the investors of the world. We are looking at a country that is very integrated and very synergic, and a country that is actually setting and driving trends, rather than following them.

Questions:

1. Which country is talked about here?

2. What does "integrated and synergic" mean?

3. Why do we say China is a country that is actually setting and driving trends, rather than following them?

● China's cultural heritage and identity is a composition of over 5000 years of global integration. What is Chinese culture? China has had an incredible history of different countries and cultures coming through from the Silk Road, from Mongolia. It's been constantly reinventing itself. China is the original melting pot of cultures. There are so many motifs of Chinese culture, architecture and design.

Questions:

1. What is Chinese cultural heritage and identity composed of?

2. What is Chinese culture according to the author?

3. What's the meaning of "motifs" and can you give us any examples?

● Through four decades of economic opening and up global connectivity, economic prosperity has come to China. Starvation is no longer a problem in most Chinese cities, but Chinese people are not happier than before. With the accumulation of wealth, their anxiety level rises instead. It's not just China, but all countries of the world. You need materialism, but materialism alone is not enough. You also need spirituality, you need culture.

Questions:

1. How long has China been performing economic opening up and global connectivity?

2. Why are Chinese people not happier than before?

3. What do we need to combat anxiety after economic prosperity has come to China?

● Five years, let alone a decade ago, China was associated with cheap manufacturing. The West believed that China would for long remain essentially defined by imitation, unable to match the West's capacity for innovation. But China has proven itself to have an impressively innovative economy.

Questions:

1. What was China associated with five or ten years ago?
2. What did the West believe about China's manufacturing?
3. What has China proven about its economy?

● Perhaps the clearest demonstration of China's growing influence has been the Belt and Road Initiative—a global network of Chinese-financed highways, railways, ports and energy infrastructure, launched in 2013. The ambition is no less than the transformation of Eurasia, home to more than 60% of the world's population. More than 140 countries, overwhelmingly from the developing world, have now signed up; and the great majority were represented by their leaders at the Belt and Road Summit held in early 2019, a level of representation no other country could match, the US included.

Questions:

1. What is the Belt and Road Initiative according to the text?
2. Why is the Belt and Road Initiative ambitious?
3. Why has the Belt and Road Summit held in early 2019 reached a level of representation no other country could match?

Part III Moral Tips

1. The beacon fire has gone higher and higher; Words from household are

worth their weight in gold.

烽火连三月，家书抵万金。

——杜甫

2. Be man of men while you are alive; Be soul of souls e'en though you're dead! Think of Xiang Yu who'd not survive. His men, whose blood for him was shed.

生当作人杰，死亦为鬼雄。至今思项羽，不肯过江东。

——李清照

3. In the entire course of history, the liberation and progress of women have been indispensable to the liberation and progress of mankind. Since its inception, the Communist Party of China (CPC) has been struggling for women's liberation and gender equality.

纵观历史，没有妇女解放和进步，就没有人类解放和进步。中国共产党从诞生之日起就把实现妇女解放、促进男女平等写在奋斗的旗帜上。

——《平等　发展　共享：新中国 70 年妇女事业的发展与进步》

4. Under the leadership of the CPC, the past few generations of women have contributed greatly to social construction, reform, and development. As the Chinese nation is rising and growing richer and stronger, Chinese women's social status has undergone enormous changes. As masters of the nation, women now can find the best ways to fulfill themselves while gaining increasing senses of achievement, happiness, and safety, as witnessed by the historic accomplishments they've made so far.

在中国共产党领导下，一代又一代妇女为中国的建设、改革与发展开拓进取、贡献力量。在中华民族从站起来、富起来到强起来的伟大飞跃中，中国妇女地位发生了翻天覆地的巨大变化。亿万妇女主人翁的地位更加彰显，半边天力量充分释放，获得感、幸福感、安全感与日俱增。中国妇女事业取得举世瞩目的历史性成就。

——《平等　发展　共享：新中国 70 年妇女事业的发展与进步》

5. China has maintained an international outlook. China gives attention to the modernization of the world. The aim is to build a community with a shared future and to develop a new type of human civilization through international cooperation, calling for and promoting the joint construction of the Belt and Road Initiative, and pledging to reduce carbon emissions. China has acted as a responsible and broad-minded major country.

中国一直保持着国际视野。中国对世界的现代化给予关注。目的是通过国际合作，呼吁和推动"一带一路"倡议的共同建设，承诺减少碳排放，建立一个拥有共同未来的社区，发展新型的人类文明。中国作为一个负责任的、心胸宽广的大国，已经行动起来。

Part IV Vocabulary Treasure

1. **momentous** *adj.* (of a decision, event, or change) of great importance or significance, especially in its bearing on the future
The five years since the 19th National Congress have been truly **momentous** and extraordinary.
十九大以来的五年，是极不寻常、极不平凡的五年。

2. **heritage** *n.* property that is or may be inherited; an inheritance
Xi underlined the need for solid measures to protect intangible cultural **heritage**, meet the people's increasing demand for intellectual and cultural life and boost their cultural confidence and strength.
习近平强调，需要采取扎实的措施保护非物质文化遗产，满足人民群众日益增长的知识文化生活需求，增强人民的文化自信和实力。

3. **determination** *n.* firmness of purpose; resoluteness
With great effort and **determination**, we have steadily advanced socialism with Chinese characteristics in the new era.
以奋发有为的精神把新时代中国特色社会主义不断推向前进。

4. flourish   *v.*   to grow or develop successfully

Only by taking root in the rich historical and cultural soil of the country and the nation can the truth of Marxism **flourish** here.

只有植根本国、本民族历史文化沃土，马克思主义真理之树才能根深叶茂。

5. initiative   *n.*   a proposal

Let's Exercise for Better Health **Initiative**, through which we hope to showcase the tenacious spirit of athletes, and promote the joy of the sport.

我们希望通过"让我们为健康而运动"的倡议来展示运动员的顽强精神，并促进运动的乐趣。

Part V   Language Practice

1. Translate the following paragraph into English.

中华民族的传统文化博大精深，源远流长。早在 2000 多年前，就产生了儒家学说、道家学说，以及其他许多中国思想史上有地位的学说和学派。中华民族传统文化有许多宝贵财富，比如强调仁爱、群体、天下为公，以及代代相传的吃苦耐劳、勤俭持家、尊师重教的传统美德。所有这些，对国家、社会和家庭都起到了重要的维系和调节作用，对个人成长和发展具有重要意义。

2. Critical Thinking

This part is to improve the critical thinking ability by writing a composition.

Direction: Write a composition on the topic: Chinese Dream, My Dream.

The composition is based on the following information, and it is at least 120 words.

> ➢ **What is Chinese Dream?**
> ➢ **What is your dream?**
> ➢ **How to combine them?**

Part VI Further Reading

Ren Shasha's job requires her to play many roles. She may need to play the part of a hotel receptionist, a passer-by, or even a couple with her colleague. However, these roles are all unrelated to the acting profession. They are instead a crucial part of her job as a border policewoman fighting drugs.

She once intercepted a vehicle and seized heroin from the spare tire. Unexpectedly, she also found a handgun and a dozen rounds of ammunition just below the driver's seat.

"The drug dealers were ready to bend over and reach for the gun," recalled Ren.

"I was really afraid afterward. I could not bear to think about the potential consequences if they were arrested just a few seconds late." But all she could think of at that moment was catching the criminals and ensuring that they faced the full consequences of their actions under the law.

Born in 1993 in Nanchong, Southwest China's Sichuan province, Ren had dreamed of joining the army since she was a little girl, and she finally made it in 2012. She became an anti-drug policewoman in 2016.

Undoubtedly one of the most dangerous jobs in peacetime, the anti-drug operation is a path that few are willing to tread, and for females, this path is even more daunting.

"In the fight against drugs, there is no concept of 'the man goes first and the woman comes later'," Ren said.

In 2018, Ren had a chance of retirement, and her parents wanted her to return to Sichuan, but she "willfully" chose to work at the Mukang border checkpoint in Southwest China's Yunnan province, which is the first barrier stopping drugs from flowing from the border to the Chinese mainland.

"Because in all my years of fighting drugs, I've seen too many people and too many families destroyed by drugs. I once saw a gaunt, middle-aged woman with four children, one of whom a toddler who didn't even have shoes. All because their father exhausted all his money on drugs," she said.

"I want to do everything in my power to stop the spread of drugs, apprehend more drug-related criminals, and restore a clean society."

In May 2022, the usually calm Ren was caught off guard after she was diagnosed with "thyroid cancer".

She had a choice between surgery or conservative treatment, but if she accepted the latter, she would have to stop her intensive work and move to an in-house position. Ren finally decided to undergo surgery in June 2022 and returned to her post in September.

After returning, a drug dealer openly threatened her physically during the interrogation.

"I've kept you in my mind, and you'd better not give me a chance to get out, or I'll kill you," the suspect threatened.

"I'm not even afraid of cancer, let alone a drug dealer," Ren calmly replied.

The fact of the matter is that Ren has been walking on the brink of life and death since the day when she decided to become an anti-drug policewoman.

So far, Ren has participated in the seizure of more than 130 drug cases, arrested more than 140 suspects, and seized more than 400 kilograms of various drugs, winning herself the honor of China's female role models.

Together with their male colleagues, policewomen like Ren have fought bravely on the front lines of fighting drugs, and showed no fear.

They exemplify strong characteristics of women such as selflessness and fearlessness, taking responsibility as a demonstration of women's strength. They are also children, wives, and mothers, and the epitome of millions of women.

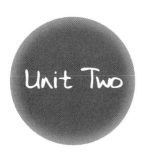

Unit Two

Virtuous Habits

Part I   Pre-Reading Task

On Aug 12, CCTV exposed several Chinese hosts who were pretending to eat large amounts of food while on camera, but actually later threw it away.

To discourage this practice, many video and live-streaming platforms, including Douyin, Kuaishou and Bilibili, have removed videos that show food waste and have promoted messages to "stop food waste and eat reasonably".

In June 2020, the United Nations warned that the world is on the verge of the worst food crisis in 50 years.

According to the Food and Agriculture Organization of the United Nations, about a third of the world's food—1.3 billion tons—is wasted every year. In China alone, 50 million tons of food ends up in landfills every year, according to *Beijing News*.

Recently, campaigns against food waste have been further promoted. In August, President Xi Jinping stressed the need for safeguarding food security and halting food waste.

According to *China Daily*, restaurants and catering associations in more than 18 provinces and all 4 municipal cities have issued guidelines to control food waste.

Meanwhile, new laws are also being considered, according to *China Daily*. "We will make new laws that give clear instructions on avoiding food waste," said

Zhang Guilong from the Legislative Affairs Committee of the National People's Congress. The instructions will be detailed in every part of food production, purchasing, storage, transportation, processing and consumption, according to Zhang.

Questions:

1. Do you think it is right to remove videos that show food waste? Why?
2. Do you think that the public media should be responsible to promote the traditional Chinese culture? Why?
3. Can you find any lines that are connected with the value of thrift from the Chinese classic literature, e.g. *Confucius*, *Tao Te Ching*?

Part II   Reading Task

● The paradox is that every day we get two sets of messages at odds with each other. One is the "permissive" perspective, "Buy, spend, get it now. You need this!" The other we could call an "upright" message, which urges us, "Work hard and save. Suspend your desires. Avoid luxuries. Control your appetite for more than you truly need."

Questions:

1. How do you understand the phrase "work hard and save"?
2. What are the "core socialist values"?
3. How to put the "core socialist values" into practice from your view?

● What happens as we take in these contradictory but explicit messages? What are the psychological and social consequences of this campaign to control our spending habits? ... On the other hand, a little voice inside us echoes those upright messages: "Watch out, take stock of your life, don't let your attention get scattered. Postpone your desires. Don't fall into debt. Wait! Retain control over your own life. It will make you stronger."

Campus loan generally refers to a loan given to a college student on the campus, but it is in essence a private loan. Internet lenders, most of whom are loan sharks, offer such loans to students who need the money to meet their college and other expenses.

Questions:
1. How do you understand the phrase "take stock of your life"?
2. What are the dangers of campus loan?
3. How do you relieve the financial burden in the university, to gain the scholarship or to do the part time job?

● Anyway, many of the skills you need as a successful student can be applied to your finances. Consider your financial well-being as a key ingredient of your university education as money worries are extremely stressful and distracting. They can make you feel terrible and hinder your ability to focus on your prime objective: successfully completing your education.

Questions:
1. Will money worries become one of the reasons that distract your university education? Why?
2. How do you complete your education in the university?
3. What is a successful education?

● Minimalism is about getting rid of excess stuff and keeping only what you need. Minimalist living, in simplest terms, is to live with as less as possible, mentally and physically until you achieve peace of mind. Results that ensue are less stress, more time, and increased happiness. Minimalists like to say that they're living more meaningfully more deliberately, and that the minimalist lifestyle allows them to focus on what's more important in life: friends, hobbies, travel, experiences.

Questions:

1. What are the more important things in your life besides material stuff?
2. How do you understand the phrase "achieve peace of mind"?
3. Do you think self-control and self-discipline can also increase happiness?

● All this will help you become an educated consumer and saver. As you learn to balance spending and saving, you will become the captain of your own ship, steering your life in a successful and productive direction through the choppy waters.

Questions:

1. How do you understand the phrase "balance spending and saving"?
2. How can you overcome the obstacles through life's dangerous sea?
3. What's a successful direction?

Part III   Moral Tips

1. There is delight in plain food and water while pillowing the head on the arm. I would keep ill-gotten wealth and rank as far away as floating cloud.

饭疏食，饮水，曲肱而枕之，乐亦在其中矣。不义而富且贵，于我如浮云。

——《论语》

2. I have three treasures to hold and preserve: humanity, frugality and humility.

我有三宝，持而保之：一曰慈，二曰俭，三曰不敢为天下先。

——《道德经》

3. This is a way of life for a man of virtue: to cultivate his character by keeping a peaceful mind, and nourish his morality by thrifty living. Without being pure, a bright ambition is in vain; without being indifferent, a far-off goal is no gain.

夫君子之行，静以修身，俭以养德。非淡泊无以明志，非宁静无以致远。

——诸葛亮

4. Young people shall nurture and practise core socialist values, and guard against wrong ideas such as money worship, hedonism, extreme individualism and historical nihilism.

青年应当培养和践行社会主义核心价值观，防范金钱崇拜、享乐主义、极端个人主义、历史虚无主义等错误观念。

5. To all our young people, you should have firm ideals and convictions, aim high, and have your feet firmly on the ground. You should ride the waves of your day; and in the course of realizing the Chinese Dream, fulfill your youthful dreams, and write a vivid chapter in your tireless endeavors to serve the interests of the people.

广大青年要坚定理想信念，志存高远，脚踏实地，勇做时代的弄潮儿，在实现中国梦的生动实践中放飞青春梦想，在为人民利益的不懈奋斗中书写人生华章！

Part IV   Vocabulary Treasure

1. **morality** *n.* concern with the distinction between good and evil or right and wrong; right or good conduct

We will continue the civic **morality** campaign, carry forward traditional Chinese virtues, foster strong family ties, values and traditions, and raise the intellectual and moral standards of minors.

我们将继续实施公民道德建设工程，弘扬中华传统美德，加强家庭家教家风建设，加强和改进未成年人思想道德建设。

2. **frugality**   *n.*   the quality of being frugal, sparing, thrifty, prudent or economical in the consumption of consumable resources such as food, time or money, and avoiding waste, lavishness or extravagance

We will foster an ethos of work, enterprise, dedication, creativity, and **frugality** throughout society and cultivate new trends and new customs for our times.

我们将在全社会弘扬劳动精神、奋斗精神、奉献精神、创造精神、勤俭节约精神，培育时代新风新貌。

3. **conviction**   *n.*   a strong belief that is not likely to change, or the strong feeling that your beliefs are right

Xi, general secretary of the Communist Party of China Central Committee, called on children to study hard, firm up their ideals and **convictions** and develop strong bodies and minds to get prepared for realizing the Chinese Dream of national rejuvenation.

习近平总书记希望广大少年儿童刻苦学习知识，坚定理想信念，磨练坚强意志，锻炼强健体魄，为实现中华民族伟大复兴的中国梦时刻准备着。

4. **milestone**   *n.*   an important event in the development or history of something or in someone's life

2020 will be a year of **milestone** significance. We will finish building a moderately prosperous society in all respects and realize the first centenary goal.

2020年是具有里程碑意义的一年。我们将全面建成小康社会，实现第一个百年奋斗目标。

5. **cradle**   *n.*   a small bed for a baby, especially one that moves from side to side

   Asia is home to one of the earliest human settlements and an important **cradle** of human civilizations.

   亚洲是人类最早的定居地之一，也是人类文明的重要发祥地。

6. **emulate**   *v.*   strive to equal or match, especially by imitating

   We will see that Party and State awards and honors play a guiding and exemplary role and that a public atmosphere prevails in which people **emulate** paragons of virtue, look up to heroes, and strive to become pioneers.

   发挥党和国家功勋荣誉表彰的精神引领、典型示范作用、推动全社会见贤思齐、崇尚英雄、争做先锋。

Part V   Language Practice

1. Translate the following paragraph into English.

不论我们国家发展到什么水平，不论人民生活改善到什么地步，艰苦奋斗、勤俭节约的思想永远不能丢。艰苦奋斗、勤俭节约，不仅是我们一路走来、发展壮大的重要保证，也是我们继往开来、再创辉煌的重要保证。

2. Critical Thinking

This part is to improve the critical thinking ability by writing a composition.

Direction: Write a composition on the topic: Extravagant Spending on College Campus.

The composition is based on the following information, and it is at least 120 words.

  ➢ **higher expenditure of college students**

  ➢ **concept of frugality**

  ➢ **my opinion**

Part VI   Further Reading

1. Save the food: Raising awareness of food waste among young Chinese (excerpt)

More than 80 percent of roughly 2,000 respondents said they are aware of food waste issues, and more than 84 percent of the Gen-Z group made it clear they were eager to reduce food waste, according to a recent poll conducted by *China Youth Daily*.

Additionally, attitudes about young people towards food waste varied. About 50 percent of survey respondents thought that young people were aware of the issue, while 23 percent thought otherwise. Specifically, respondents in second-tier Chinese cities said young people there are aware of food waste issues.

Saving food as a habit

"When I was young, my grandparents would scold me if I left food on my plate. Their generation had gone through tough times living in poverty, so they cannot accept that people don't cherish food," said Wang Feng, who works in Beijing. Influenced by his grandparents, Wang says food waste is still not a big issue among some of his friends. "It's not about being rich or poor, it's a way of life. Personally, I ask my friends how much they can have when we eat outside. Usually, everyone will eat the food, and people feel no pressure to bring any leftovers home."

"I always take the leftovers home if we eat out," said Zhou Xiao, who also lives in Beijing with her husband. With their busy lives in cities, Zhou added that she spends less time cooking and orders out more often. Half-serve orders, which have gained popularity on delivery apps, offer people like Zhou the option to reduce food waste without worrying about the portion size.

There is also a growing trend among Chinese people to serve fewer dishes at weddings and birthday banquets to reduce waste. While big portions used to be a social indicator, some are trying to cut down on the food waste. "Though some old relatives cannot understand it since they believe it's about 'face,' me and my wife agreed to cut the size and amount of our wedding dishes. It's heartbreaking to see all the untouched leftovers get thrown away," said Hailu Wang, a groom-to-be in Shanghai.

2. Money-saving lifestyle hailed by young 'frugal' Chinese

"As a painter, I want to study the masters' works in detail, but they are too pricey. The cheapest art book is around 200 yuan, and you always have to wait for the popular ones in the library to be free. So, I choose to look for used books." Wang Shu'ai, a 28-year-old oil painting student, has been a fan of buying and trading art books on Xianyu, a popular Chinese second-hand goods exchange platform, for more than four years. Wang is one of an expanding group of young Chinese who have been pursuing a thrifty and green lifestyle by methods such as bringing their own bags instead of plastics ones while shopping and collecting coupons. In China, they have a new name "Koukouzu," or "the young frugal Chinese."

"Garish advertising and some lip-service to some e-commerce shops hold less attraction for today's young Chinese. What truly grabs their attention are tangible benefits when it comes to price and the quality of goods," Ding Daoshi, a independent internet analyst, told the *Global Times*.

Price and quality

After four years on Xianyu, Wang has developed a knack for saving money while still finding the books she needs. Her most successful purchase was a collection of works by Francis Bacon bought from a Shanghai seller. The collection was 399 yuan on Taobao, but she bought it for only around 150 yuan, Wang told the *Global Times*. Eventually, Wang decided to start her own tiny business selling high-quality second-hand books. She also began renting books to her classmates.

The second-hand market, both online and offline, is a channel for young Chinese to save money, so services for trading in used goods for new ones and exchanging unused items has seen success. Data from JD.com shows that in the first quarter of 2022, the number of users participating in mobile phone trade-in increased by nearly five times year-on-year. In the meanwhile, young users aged 18—35 accounted for 60 percent of people who have once used trade-in services.

Wan, a 27-year-old Wuhan resident, told the Global Times that when buying a new phone she was able to save herself 500 yuan by trading in her old one through a second-hand service at the store. She also decided to get some money back by putting some furniture she had bought to decorate her rented apartment up for sale online before moving back to Wuhan from Beijing. "Why not? I get material benefits and at the same time, these items will not be wasted, which is also good for the environment," Wan told the *Global Times*.

For these young people, saving money does not mean having to sacrifice their quality of life. They lay equal stress on both price and the quality of the items they get in return. A report on new consumption methods of Chinese youth by Beijing Normal University said that 57.9 percent of young people care about price and among them, 62.6 percent put equal value on quality.

Waste not, want not

More young people are also focusing on spending their money on more environmentally friendly products to do their part to protect the environment. The lifestyle begins with actions such as not ordering takeout, bringing their own bags instead of using plastic ones from the supermarket and bringing their own coffee cups to coffee shops.

Inside a small alley in a Beijing city center stands an unremarkable store that focuses on zero waste products and lifestyles, The Bulk House. On its shelves are a series of products made from eco-friendly, biodegradable or second-hand materials. And the shop owner tries her best to minimize the use of packaging.

The shop attracts young people with the concept of minimalism. Hu, a costumer who works as a consultant, told the *Global Times* that she bought a shopping bag there and has been using it at the supermarket for the past three years. "It may not seem like a big deal, but the money spent on plastic bags adds up over the years and the negative impact on the environment goes beyond numbers." Young Chinese today are breaking the stereotype that young people are all about spending money on unnecessary items, without sacrificing quality of life or the environment.

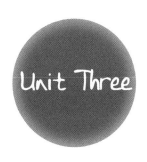

Unit Three

Value Guidance

Part I   Pre-Reading Task

A heartwarming letter written by Yuan Longping, the agronomist known as "the father of hybrid rice", has caught people's eyes as the nation is mourning over his passing away. In 2010, at the age 80, Yuan wrote this letter in memory of his late mother, Hua Jing, and many are deeply touched by its sincerity.

In the letter, entitled "The Rice is Ripe, Mom", Yuan recalled the old days with his mother in Anjiang town in Central China's Hunan province, where he devoted himself to the study of hybrid rice. His mother was buried there in 1989.

Born in a wealthy merchant family in Yangzhou, eastern China's Jiangsu province, Hua Jing was well educated and open-minded. She taught Yuan English and the thoughts of Nietzsche when he was very young. Having never worked in the fields, Hua moved to Anjiang town to support her son's family and research.

"Mom, the rice is ripe and I come back to Anjiang to see you. Every time when I was able to deliver a speech to the audiences from around the world or take a prize in my study, I always thought of you. You made me who I am. People say I've changed the world with one tiny rice seed but mom, I know you sowed the seed in me when I was a little boy."

Questions:

1. What do you know about Yuan Longping and his mother Hua Jiang?

2. Born in a wealthy family in the metropolis of Yangzhou, Yuan Longping and his mother were devoted to the fields of Anjiang town. What do you think of their choice? What kind of values and virtues do you learn from them?

3. What are Yuan Longping's contributions to people's health?

Part II   Reading Task

● Yet I feel nothing more than a passing whim to attain the material things so many other people have. My 1999 car shows the wear and tear of 105,000 miles. But it is still dependable. My apartment is modest, but quiet and relaxing. My clothes are well suited to my work, which is primarily outdoors. My minimal computer needs can be met at the library.

Questions:

1. Do you think attaining the material things is "nothing more than a passing whim"?

2. What are the similarities between the author and Yan Hui in *the Analects of Confucius* in attaining the material things?

3. How did the Master praise "the virtue of Yan Hui"? Do you agree?

● I've enjoyed exceptionally good health for 53 years. It's not just that I've been illness-free, it's that I feel vigorous and spirited. Exercising is actually fun for me. I look forward to long, energizing walks. And I love the "can do" attitude that follows.

Questions:

1. How does the author define "good health"?
2. What is WHO's definition of "good health"?
3. What does "can do" attitude mean? Do you think exercising brings "can do" attitude to people?

● I'm continually surprised at the insights that come through my writing process. And talking with so many interesting writer friends is one of my main sources of enjoyment.

But there is one vital area of my life where I am not so well off. In a society that spends so much emotional energy on the pursuit of possessions, I feel out of place.

Questions:

1. What does "the pursuit of possessions" refer to?
2. Do you think our society "spends so much emotional energy on the pursuit of possessions"? Why or why not?
3. What is Confucius's attitude towards "the pursuit of possessions"?

● But I'm happy to live without one. In fact, not being focused on material goods feels quite natural to me. There are many people throughout the world who would consider my lifestyle to be affluent.

Questions:

1. Do you sometimes feel the pressure to purchase some popular material goods?
2. What is the author's lifestyle? Do you think his lifestyle is affluent?
3. What kind of lifestyle do you think is healthy and worth pursuing?

● Near the end of the year, when I put on the Salvation Army's red apron, something changes inside me. Instead of feeling out of place economically, I begin to feel a genuine sense of belonging. As I ring my bell, people stop to share their personal stories of how much it meant to be helped when they were going through a rough time. People helping people is something I feel deeply connected to.

Questions:

1. How do you understand "a sense of belonging" in the text? Do you think "having a sense of belonging" will benefit people's mental health?

2. What does the author mean by saying "People helping people is something I feel deeply connected to"?

3. How do a paid part-time job and a voluntary charity work benefit college students respectively?

Part III　Moral Tips

1. The Master said, "Admirable indeed was the virtue of Hui! With a single bamboo dish of rice, a single gourd dish of drink, and living in his mean narrow lane, while others could not have endured the distress, he did not allow his joy to be affected by it. Admirable indeed was the virtue of Hui!"

子曰:"贤哉，回也！一箪食，一瓢饮，在陋巷，人不堪其忧，回也不改其乐。贤哉，回也！"

——《论语》

2. The Master said, "If the search for riches is sure to be successful, though I should become a groom with whip in hand to get them, I will do so. As the search may not be successful, I will follow after that which I love."

子曰："富而可求也，虽执鞭之士，吾亦为之。如不可求，从吾所好。"

——《论语》

3. Care for my own aged parents and extend the same care to the aged parents of others; love my own young children and extend the same love to the children of others.

老吾老，以及人之老；幼吾幼，以及人之幼。

——《孟子》

4. A strong determination to get the best out of life, a keen desire to enjoy what one has, and no regrets if one fails: this is the secret of the Chinese genius for contentment.

一个强烈的决心，以摄取人生至善至美；一股殷热的欲望，以享乐一身之所有，但倘令命该无福可享，则亦不怨天尤人。这是中国人"知足"的精义。

——林语堂

5. The effect of physical education is to strengthen the muscles and bones, thus increasing knowledge, regulating emotions, and strengthening the will. Muscles and bones are our body; knowledge, emotion and will are our heart. With comfort body and mind, you are in a good state.

体育之效，至于强筋骨，因而增知识，因而调感情，因而强意志。筋骨者，吾人之身；知识，感情，意志者，吾人之心。身心皆适，是谓俱泰。

——毛泽东

Part IV   Vocabulary Treasure

1. **attain**   *v.*   to gain with effort
We had multiple targets to **attain**, like ensuring stable growth and

preventing risks; multiple tasks to complete, like promoting economic and social development; and multiple relationships to handle, like that between short-term and long-term interests.

实现稳增长、防风险等多重目标，完成经济社会发展等多项任务，处理好当前与长远等多种关系。

2. **cherish** *v.* be fond of; be attached to

We should make efforts to ensure coexistence between man and nature, cherish the environment as we **cherish** our own lives, respect and protect nature, and safeguard the irreplaceable planet Earth.

我们应该坚持人与自然共生共存的理念，像对待生命一样对待生态环境，对自然心存敬畏，尊重自然、顺应自然、保护自然，共同保护不可替代的地球家园。

3. **affluent** *adj.* having an abundant supply of money or possessions of value

Diabetes—long perceived as a disease of the **affluent**—is on the rise everywhere and is now most common in developing countries.

糖尿病长久以来被认为是富贵病，目前在全球呈上升趋势，现在在发展中国家最为常见。

4. **tangible** *adj.* perceptible by the senses especially the sense of touch

The UN should aim at problem solving and move toward **tangible** outcomes as it advances security, development and human rights in parallel.

联合国要以解决问题为出发点，以可视成果为导向，平衡推进安全、发展、人权。

5. **emotional** *adj.* connected with people's feelings

Other apps have the ability to personalize healthy living suggestions based on the users' location and self-reported characteristics such as health status, **emotional** well-being and physical environment.

另外有一些应用程序可以根据用户的地理位置和自身的特点（例如健康状况、情感状态、外部环境），给用户提出个性化的健康建议。

6. **minimal** *adj.*　very small in quantity, value, or degree

   Shandong Cuisine is characterized by its emphasis on aroma, freshness, crispness and tenderness and the use of **minimal** fat.

   鲁菜的特点是强调香、鲜、脆、嫩，以及使用脂肪含量尽可能少的食材。

7. **go through**　pursue to a conclusion or bring to a successful issue

   We need to learn from comparing long history cycles, and see the change in things through the subtle and minute. We need to foster new opportunities amidst crises, open up new horizons on a shifting landscape, and pool great strength to **go through** difficulties and challenges.

   我们要善于从历史长周期比较分析中进行思考，又要善于从细微处洞察事物的变化，在危机中育新机、于变局中开新局，凝聚起战胜困难和挑战的强大力量。

Part V　Language Practice

1. Translate the following paragraph into English.

　　我为什么要对青年讲讲社会主义核心价值观这个问题？是因为青年的价值取向决定了未来整个社会的价值取向，而青年又处在价值观形成和确立的时期，抓好这一时期的价值观养成十分重要。这就像穿衣服扣扣子一样，如果第一粒扣子扣错了，剩余的扣子都会扣错。人生的扣子从一开始就要扣好。"凿井者，起于三寸之坎，以就万仞之深。"青年要从现在做起、从自己做起，使社会主义核心价值观成为自己的基本遵循，并身体力行大力将其推广到全社会去。

2. Critical Thinking

This part is to improve the critical thinking ability by writing a composition.

Direction: Write a composition on the topic: Can living simply make life less stressful and more fulfilling? The composition is based on the following information, and it is at least 120 words.

> ➢ **embrace a simple and healthy lifestyle**
>
> ➢ **get rid of the excess of life and acquire self-fulfillment**
>
> ➢ **my opinion**

Part VI Further Reading

1. Mountain teacher opens art's door to left-behind kids

The Xiansheng School of Art and Craft is a non-profit organization founded by Chinese artist Xin Wangjun. It is designed to help left-behind children in China's remote areas embrace their artistic spirits.

In 2016, Xin established the first School of Art and Craft in frontier Lianghe county, southwest China's Yunnan province. Lianghe county is an agricultural area lying dozens of kilometers from the Sino-Myanmar border area.

A lot of young Chinese people move to big cities, leaving the elderly and children at home. Feng Yuqiong, 22, is different. She is an art teacher at the School of Art and Craft. "School of Art and Craft is a place fulfilling my childhood dream," she said.

In September 2017, Feng went to the mountains by motorcycle to teach art to 60 students at Qingping primary school in Mangdong town, Lianghe county of Dehong prefecture in Yunnan province.

Only seven teachers taught lessons in the school. None specialized in art or music. If she weren't there teaching, the art classroom would have been locked up.

Feng prepared many songs for students to sing at her first class. To her delight and surprise, all the children joined her in singing *Flying Worm.*

She wants the children to feel happy, free, and love nature, while opening their imaginations. By teaching the children to paint by rubbing and printing leaves on paper, she wants them to learn that getting in touch with nature is something to be proud of.

She sang the song "You Are My Sunshine" to all the children because they light up her days, giving her the courage and will to keep teaching in the mountains. "Their smiling faces are the best sugar I have ever eaten," said Feng.

She fondly recalls the environment of her childhood, when she lived in her grandmother's house on the mountain. She caught crabs and fish in the river and fed ducks. Nature remains her source of inspiration. She is especially good at painting flowers and plants.

Feng was ill during her primary school years. When she was a high school sophomore, she got caught up in an accident and spent time in a coma. She was depressed after this, and found communicating with others difficult.

However, embracing painting and nature helped her feel stronger and everything took a positive turn when she joined the School of Art and Craft as a volunteer teacher. The first painting she created in the School of Art and Craft was later exhibited in a small town in France.

In the future, she hopes to invite local high school students to clean up the School of Art and Craft and enhance the sense of community among youngsters.

Feng drew a door of time travel on the wall, and hopes to lead the children through it. She is determined to continue working at the School of Art and Craft because only by doing so can she make a difference to the education of the locals.

2. Sun Simiao: A Pioneer in TCM Development

Sun Simiao, a pioneer of the comprehensive and systematic study of Traditional Chinese Medicine (TCM), is revered as the "Medicine God" or the "King of Medicine" by Chinese people. He was a great medical expert of China in the Tang Dynasty (618—907).

Sun is said to have studied hard and mastered several Chinese classics by the age of 20. He did extensive research on ancient medical classics, and according to historical records, in the history of TCM, he had particularly innovative views on medical ethics, gynecology, pediatrics, acupuncture, and other topics. Sun held noble medical ethics in high regard, and his perspective on medical ethics was pivotal in the history of Chinese medicine. From his point of view, the doctor's sole responsibility is to relieve patients' pain without being influenced by a desire for reward, such as financial gain, fame, or favors bestowed upon them. Patients should be treated fairly, regardless of their rank, wealth, or other eternal factors, said Sun. In his well-known book *Qianjin Yaofang*, he proposed that a good doctor should place equal emphasis on medical ethics and skills.

Sun's experience with herb formulas and knowledge of medicine was documented in *Qianjin Yaofang*. The book presented life-saving remedies as well as case studies on acupuncture, massage, diet, and exercise. Sun wrote a second well-known book, *Qianjin Yifang*, as supplement to his earlier work. Both of the books are still in print today. His writings focused on the treatment of women and children, with special volumes devoted to female disorders (and pregnancy), infant diseases and breastfeeding.

Sun's research on health care was highly insightful. In terms of his overall health philosophy, he believed that people should combine massage therapies, physical exercise, and breathing exercises. He advocated disease prevention, emphasizing the importance of "caution in a speech before sleep" and "moderation in eating".

Sun was described as a "magnificent teacher of hundreds of generations" by Li Shimin, Emperor of the Tang Dynasty. Some of Sun's revolutionary ideas can be used as a reference for current medical development, and his nurturing method for health still remains popular among people of all ages.

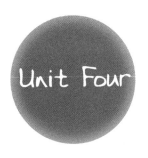

Belief Persistence

Part I   Pre-Reading Task

While wearing a mask in this new norm might pose just a slight inconvenience to most people, this new practice has inadvertently created another hurdle for hearing impaired people like Cai Zhengjun, who runs a design studio in Shanghai that helps imbue self-confidence in their hearing-impaired staff while honing their creative skills.

Cai lost his hearing when he was just 18 months old, the result of a high fever and an allergic reaction to the penicillin which was prescribed to him. Having lived most of his life in near complete silence, the 35-year-old is well aware of the emotional baggage that comes with this condition.

He recalls having suffered from self-esteem issues when he was a child, and how attempting to communicate with others became a daunting affair.

Fortunately, his parents were determined to see their son equipped with the necessary life skills needed to lead a normal life.

Today, Cai's role has changed from a silent observer in life to a source of empowerment for his fellow hearing-impaired peers.

At his art studio LFORU, only deaf individuals can be found working behind the counter. Every person here is free to create whatever he or she desires.

"I want my colleagues to do whatever they like. I believe this is how they can produce their best work," he explained.

"Hearing-impaired people also have their advantages. They tend to be more focused and serious about matters," he added.

"Sometimes, we're able to do things even better than others, but it takes a lot more effort for us because of this communication barrier."

Questions:

1. Do you support the disabled to work in public places? Why or why not?

2. In your opinion, what are the obstacles to success for the disabled? How to overcome these obstacles?

3. "Sometimes, we're able to do things even better than others, but it takes a lot more effort for us because of this communication barrier." What's your opinion about the words of Cai? And what do you think you can do for the disabled like them?

Part II Reading Task

• Wherever he flew was with a keen eye for detail and the free spirit of his mother's love. His dad, on the other hand, was not a dreamer. Bert Stone was a hard-core realist. He believed in hard work and sweat. His motto: If you want something, work for it!

Questions:

1. How do you think the different loves between parents affect the children? What have you learnt from your parents? You may give an example or some details.

2. Have you ever worked for something you want? Share with us your experience.

3. Do you have a motto? What 's it? How will you put it into practice?

● From the age of 14, Michael did just that. He began a very careful training program. He worked out every other day with weightlifting, with some kind of running work on alternate day. ... Michael's dedication, determination and discipline was a coach's dream.

Questions:

1. What's the meaning of the last sentence according to your understanding?
2. What can you learn from Michael's experience?
3. How do you understand dedication, determination and discipline? Do you think which one is the most important? Explain your reasons.

● All of Michael's vaults today seemed to be the reward for his hard work... He seemed unaware of the fact that he had just beaten his personal best by three inches and that he was one of the final two competitors in the pole-vaulting event at the National Junior Olympics.

Questions:

1. The passage says Michael Stone seemed unaware of his achievement at the moment. Why? Explain how you comprehend his reaction.
2. What do you think is the reason why Michael, as a blind teenager, could succeed? And imagine what kind of difficulties or obstacles he has met.
3. Do you think hard work must bring us success? Why or why not?

● He knew it was time for his final jump. Since the other vaulter had fewer misses, Michael needed to clear this vault to win. A miss would get him second place. Nothing to be ashamed of, but Michael would not allow himself the thought of not winning first place.

Questions:

1. Since winning second place is nothing to be ashamed of, why didn't Michael allow himself to think of not winning first place? Is it contradictory? Why?

2. From these words, what can you learn about Michael? What kind of characters may he have?

3. Do you agree with "Friendship First, Competition Second"? What's your opinion about the place in a competition?

● With all the media attention and sponsorship possibilities, Michael's life would never be the same again. It wasn't just because he won the National Junior Olympics and set a new world record. And it wasn't because he had just increased his personal best by $9\frac{1}{2}$ inches. It was simply because Michael Stone is blind.

Questions:

1. Are you shocked by the ending that Michael Stone is blind? What's your feeling and how do you think Michael's story will affect you and your life?

2. The passage says, "Michael's life would never be the same again." What changes do you think would happen to Michael Stone? Is it beneficial or not? Why?

3. There's a saying in China "Fame portends trouble for men just as fattening does for pigs." What's your idea about it?

Part III   Moral Tips

1. Long, long had been my road and far, far was the journey;

I will go up and down to seek my heart's desire.

路漫漫其修远兮，吾将上下而求索。

——屈原

2. When Heaven is about to place a great burden on a man, it always tests his resolution first, exhausts his body and makes him suffer great hardships, frustrates his efforts to recover from mental lassitude. Then Heaven toughens his nature and makes good his deficiencies.

天将降大任于是人也，必先苦其心志，劳其筋骨，饿其体肤，空乏其身，行拂乱其所为，所以动心忍性，曾益其所不能。

——《孟子》

3. Few things are impossible in themselves; and it is often for want of will, rather than of means, that man fails to succeed. (La Rocheforcauld)

事情很少有根本做不成的；其所以做不成，与其说是条件不够，不如说是由于决心不够。

——拉·罗切福考尔德

4. Pursue your object, be it what it will, steadily and indefatigably.

不管追求什么目标，都应坚持不懈。

5. There are no secrets to success. It is the result of preparation, hard work, and learning from failure.

成功没有诀窍。它是筹备、苦干，以及在失败中汲取教训的结果。

Part IV   Vocabulary Treasure

1. effort   *n.*   use of physical or mental energy, hard work

Olympism seeks to create a way of life based on the joy of **effort**, the educational value of setting a good example, social responsibility and respect for universal fundamental ethical principles.

奥林匹克主义力求创造一种生活方式，这种方式让人们体会到努力的乐趣，感受到榜样带来的价值，体会到社会责任还有对基本道德准则的尊重。

2. **perseverance**   *n.*   continued effort to do or achieve something despite difficulties, failure, or opposition

The *gaokao* is an good way of selecting talent, and a high score in the exam is proof of good basic knowledge, **perseverance**, patience, and a strong ability to deal with high pressure and compete with others, according to Sun Tao, president of Vision Overseas Consulting Co, a subsidiary of New Oriental Technology and Education Group.

据新东方科技教育集团子公司远景海外咨询有限公司总裁孙涛介绍，高考是选拔人才的好办法，高分证明了良好的基础知识、毅力、耐心，以及应对高压和与他人竞争的强大能力。

3. **exertion**   *n.*   the act or an instance of exerting, especially a laborious or perceptible effort

Nothing lay ahead of us but **exertion**, struggle, and perseverance. Those who were able took advantage of the opportunities for success and happiness that presented themselves.

在我们的脑海里，只剩下了努力、奋斗、锲而不舍。为的是在机会出现时能抓住属于自己的幸福与成功。

4. **bounce back**   to start to be successful again after a difficult period, for example, after experiencing failure

My mom and godparents helped me see that your performance does not define who you are as a person. They helped me realize that it is about how you respond to difficult times that matters. You have to learn to **bounce back** from trying times in life.

妈妈和教父教母让我明白，你的表现并不能定义你是一个什么样的人。他们帮助我认识到，重要的是你如何应对困难时期。你必须学会从生活的艰难时期中恢复过来 / 卷土重来。

5. **constant** *adj.* continually recurring or continuing without interruption

There is no absolute success in the world, only **constant** progress.

世上没有绝对的成功，只有不懈的努力。

6. **struggle** *v.* to make strenuous or violent efforts in the face of difficulties or opposition

As a defensive tackle for the New England Patriots, Lawrence Guy is successful today. But he **struggled** with ADHD and other learning disabilities throughout his school days. Still, he never gave up.

作为新英格兰爱国者队的防守截锋，劳伦斯·盖伊今天取得了成功。但在他的学生时代，他一直在与多动症和其他学习障碍作斗争。尽管如此，他从未放弃。

Part V   Language Practice

1. Translate the following paragraph into English.

坚持的力量

在新年到来之时，也是最盛大网球比赛之一的澳大利亚网球公开赛的时间。其中最受欢迎的男球员之一，罗杰·费德勒（Roger Federer），已经年过三十，但他仍处于顶尖水平。球迷们希望他们的英雄享受比赛就好，并不敢奢望下一个大满贯。但是罗杰做到了，他击败了对手纳达尔（Nadal），赢得了澳大利亚公开赛。世界都为他欢呼，他们见证了这个伟大的英雄在晚年再次取得事业的成功。如果我们有梦想，永远都不会太迟。人们总是以年龄为借口，实际上，他们只是缺乏坚持，这就是他们和成功人士的区别。

2. Critical Thinking

This part is to improve the critical thinking ability by writing a composition.

Direction: Write a composition on the topic: Hardship brings out the best/worst in us. The composition is based on the following information, and it is at least 120 words.

➢ **the advantages/disadvantages of hardship**

➢ **how to deal with hardship rationally**

➢ **my opinion**

Part VI   Further Reading

1. Meet Ibrahim Hamadtou, the Paralympian who plays table tennis with his mouth and foot (excerpt)

Egypt's Ibrahim Hamadtou started Para table tennis to prove to his friend that nothing is impossible. A double arm amputee, he plays with the table tennis racquet in his mouth and serves the ball using his right foot.

Challenge accepted

The Egyptian athlete lost his arms as a result of a train accident when he was 10 years old. He still remembers the day when he first started Para table tennis nearly four decades ago.

"I tried to play a number of times until I succeeded," the athlete recalled.

But it was easier said than done.

After Hamadtou took up the sport in 1986, it took him three years to be able to play with the racquet in his mouth. He practiced by himself every day by placing a table tennis table in front of a wall.

"I trained twice a day early in the morning and late at night," he said.

Smashing it to the Paralympics

Fast forward 30 years, Hamadtou competed in his first Paralympic Games at Rio 2016 and was "dazzled" to be part of the world's third largest sporting event.

He returned to the Paralympic stage five years later at Tokyo 2020, this time, focusing more on his result and performing at his best. In addition to playing in the singles tournament, Hamadtou reached the quarterfinals in the men's team classes 6—7 tournament.

While advancing to the knockout stage is an achievement Hamadtou celebrates, he also recalls the attention he received from global media in the Japanese capital.

Unique challenges

While Hamadtou's one-of-a-kind playing style has taken him to great heights, it has also taken a toll on his body.

Before the Tokyo 2020 Games, he underwent numerous scans of his teeth and had them treated with the support of different organisations.

"It's not easy at all," Hamadtou said of his style. "It's challenging especially that my playing technique put so much pressure on my back, my legs and my teeth."

Nothing is impossible

In 2019 he created a training room, which has a table tennis table and a robot that sends the ball automatically. To develop his technique, Hamadtou is especially working on serving with his foot, mixing both long and short serves.

"Playing Para table tennis has made me a very committed person."

While Hamadtou is targeting the Paris 2024 Paralympic Games, which take place in less than 500 days, he also has ambitions outside of sports. He is envisioning a career in a new field—politics.

He wants to represent people with disabilities in Egypt and discuss their needs and rights. And as Hamadtou seeks to create change, he sees his experience in Para sports becoming a motivation for many people.

He hopes to continue that by proving that there is nothing he cannot do.

"I think I am a role model as people see how I challenge myself and how I have succeeded so they know that there is nothing called impossible," he said.

2. How the Wright Brothers' Took Off

In 1900, Wilbur and Orville Wright stood on a beach in North Carolina, twisting their hands, wrists, elbows, and arms this way and that, mimicking the seabirds that soared above them. Although the brothers' movements may have looked silly, studying bird movements enabled the Wrights to unlock the secrets of flight.

From watching buzzards and pigeons fly, Wilbur learned to control the side-to-side rocking, or roll, of a glider by designing wings that could be twisted, or warped, in flight to adjust the wingtips. Other experimenters had tried and failed to control their gliders by having the operator shift his weight. Wilbur was modest, but even he said his theory was "almost revolutionary." In 1903, the Wright brothers built and flew the world's first powered airplane capable of sustained flight. They patented their wing-warping invention in 1906.

Others Laughed

Before the Wrights' success, people in the nearby town of Kitty Hawk did not understand the brothers' work. "We couldn't help thinking they were just a pair of poor nuts," John T. Daniels later admitted. "We laughed about 'em among ourselves for a while, but we soon quit laughing and just felt sorry for 'em.... Such nice boys wasting their time playing with kites and watching the gulls fly."

Mocking anyone who dreamed of flying was common during the Wrights' time, even by scientific leaders. Rear Admiral George Melville, the United States Navy's chief engineer, wrote that the dream was "wholly unwarranted, if not absurd."

Did the naysayers discourage the Wrights? Not one bit.

Not only did they have the courage to continue their pursuits; they were also willing to sacrifice their own comfort, at least temporarily. While the Wrights camped near Kitty Hawk, the weather became so cold that the water in their washbasin froze. Orville wrote to their sister Katharine, "The wind blows in on my head, and I pull the blankets up over my head, when my feet freeze, and I reverse the process. I keep this up all night and in the morning hardly able to tell 'where I'm at' in the bedclothes." Many nights, fierce storms swept along the shore, and Orville would either be up helping Wilbur hold the tent down or lying awake "expecting to see the tent get up and fly away every minute." And the brothers often ran short of food. "Will is' most starved," Orville reported.

A Swarm of Mosquitoes

In July 1901, Orville said, mosquitoes caused the "most miserable" time of his life. The insects "came in a mighty cloud, almost darkening the sun.... They chewed us clear through our underwear and socks. Lumps began swelling up all over my body like hen's eggs." The brothers wrapped themselves in blankets to escape, but with the summer heat, "Our blankets then became unbearable. The perspiration would roll off of us in torrents. We would partly uncover and the mosquitoes would swoop down upon us in vast multitudes... Misery! Misery!"

Most people would have packed up and gone home. But the brothers' never-give-up attitude was perhaps the most important key to their success. For years, the Wright brothers persisted through lack of sleep, complicated calculations, mangled gliders, and broken ribs—working and failing, working and failing— until they finally succeeded.

"What All of Us Could Do"

To achieve what they did, they were first consumed by an idea—"afflicted" was Wilbur's word—and then stuck with it.

Mr. Daniels of Kitty Hawk put it this way: "It wasn't luck that made them fly; it was hard work and hard common sense.... I'm wondering what all of us could do if we had faith in our ideas and put all our heart and mind and energy into them like those Wright boys did!"

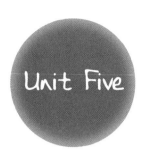

Unit Five

Aesthetics Journey

Part I Pre-Reading Task

Fifteen students from the first and second grades of No 150 Senior Middle School in Changchun, Jilin province, recently spent a week completing a copy of the painting Riverside Scene at Qingming Festival, an ancient 25-meter work by Chinese painter Zhang Zeduan in the Song Dynasty (960—1279).

The students, members of the school's painting association, used ball pens to reproduce the painting in its original proportions.

"The association was founded at the end of 2022 to allow more students to experience aesthetic education," said Duan Yingzi, an art teacher at the school. "Art education plays an important role in promoting students' cultural confidence."

Duan was surprised by the students' high level of performance.

"When I chose the famous painting for the students to copy, I believed it would be a difficult task that would require at least a month to finish," she said. "The lines of the painting are rich and complex, and so it needs great concentration and endurance to copy."

She added, "I will take students to feel the unique charm of traditional Chinese painting in different ways in the future."

A report on the development of aesthetic education was released on Nov. 26. More and more social practice in aesthetic education has made it as a way to set an example for the whole society. From rural children's choirs singing its way onto

Olympic stage to dance queens inspiring physically impaired children, dozens of Chinese stories on aesthetic education have led followers in the right direction, the report said. Those stories inspire us to go on, while unknown but outstanding teachers who make efforts to put those theories into practice can be highlighted. The seed of aesthetic education has been sown and could grow into a big tree in the near future, and what people must do is to protect it and help it grow.

Aesthetic education is one that looks to the future and integrates an appreciation of beauty from people. It gives people the ability to interpret events and experiences that are new or unpredictable, to come up with creative ideas and to break new ground—all of which are essential in an era of novel challenges and swift changes. Aesthetic education is essential to fostering talents, professionals and academicians from around the world. Art masters inspire us and lead us in the right direction, while those unknown but outstanding teachers make efforts to put those theories into practice. Aesthetic education is not a specialized form of education. It's something general for everybody. The main role of a professor is not always to give information but to engage in dialogue and appreciation of students' work. They're also in contact with students, looking for what is inside each of them and developing the qualities that each one has.

Questions:

1. What can art do? Can it cut through the wild noise of daily life? Can it connect us with basic emotions—ecstasy, anguish, desire and terror?
2. What do students benefit from the aesthetic education in the long run?
3. Can you list some ways to enhance aesthetic training?

Part II   Reading Task

● But, Lo! After the beating rain and fierce wind that had endured through the night, there yet stood out against the brick wall one ivy leaf. It was the last on the vine. Still dark green near its stem, but with its edges colored yellow, it hung bravely form a branch some twenty feet above the ground. "It is the last one," said Johnsy. "I thought it would surely fall during the night. I heard the wind. It will fall today, and I shall die at the same time."

Questions:

1. Is the ivy leaf a real ivy leaf?

2. John F. Carlson says. "Picture is a work of art, not because it is modern, nor because it is ancient, but because it is a sincere expression of human feeling". Is the "ivy leaf stood out against the brick wall" the sincere expression of human feeling? What does the "ivy leaf stood out against the brick wall" represent? Beauty? Life? Expectation? Devotion?...

3. Give more examples of the sincere expression of human feeling in art.

● The day wore away, and even through the twilight they could see the lone ivy leaf clinging to its stem against the wall. And then, with the coming of the night the north wind was again loosed. When it was light enough Johnsy, the merciless, commanded that the shad be raised. The ivy leaf was still there.

Questions:

1. Is Old Behrman a real great master who can rival these recognized great artists e.g. Rembrandt, Van Gogh...

2. Is this painting a real masterpiece? What is its greatness?

3. Comment this sentence. "All that is good in art is the expression of one soul talking to another; and is precious according to the greatness of the soul that utters it." (John Ruskin)

● "Mr. Behrman died of pneumonia today in the hospital. He was ill only two days. He was found on the morning of the first day in his room downstairs helpless with pain. His shoes and clothing were wet through and icy cold. They couldn't imagine where he had been on such a terrible night. And then they found a lantern, still lighted, and a ladder that had been dragged from its place, and some scattered brushes, and a palette with green and yellow colors mixed on it, and look out the window, dear, at the last ivy leaf on the wall. Didn't you wonder why it never fluttered or moved when the wind blew? Ah, darling, it's Behrman's masterpiece—he painted it there the night that the last leaf fell."

Questions:

1. What does the last leaf mean for Old Behrman?
2. What does the last leaf mean for Johnsy?
3. Work in pairs and talk about the power of art and the power you have gotten from art, if any.

● "You needn't get any more wine," said Johnsy, keeping her eyes fixed out the window. "There goes another. No, I don't want any soup. That leaves just four. I want to see the last one fall before it gets dark. Then I'll go, too. I'm tired of waiting. I'm tired of thinking. I want to turn my hold on everything, and go sailing down, down, just like one of those poor, tired leaves."

Questions:

1. What was, at first, Johnsy determined to do if the last ivy leaf should fall?
2. What did she decide to do when she saw the last leaf still cling to the vine after two nights' rain and wind?
3. How would Johnsy react after realizing what Mr. Behrman had done for her?

● Old Behrman was a painter who lived on the ground floor beneath them. He was past sixty and had a long white beard curling down over his chest.

Despite looking the part, Behrman was a failure in art. For forty years he had been always about to paint a masterpiece, but had never yet begun it. He earned a little by serving as a model to those young artists who could not pay the price of a professional. He drank gin to excess, and still talked of his coming masterpiece. For the rest he was a fierce little old man, who mocked terribly at softness in any one, and who regarded himself as guard dog to the two young artists in the studio above.

Questions:

1. What is your understanding of "masterpiece"? Give examples of some greatest artists and their masterpieces.
2. Why does Sue call the painted leaf Behrman's masterpiece?
3. Judging from this paragraph, what kind of person is Mr. Behrman?

Part III   Moral Tips

1. Of the *shao* music, the Master said, it was perfectly beautiful and perfectly good. Of the *wu* music, he said, it was perfectly beautiful but not perfectly good.

子谓《韶》:"尽美矣，又尽善也。"谓《武》:"尽美矣，未尽善也。"

——《论语》

2. The Master said, "in the *guanju* poem, there is joy but no immodest thoughts; sorrow but no self-injury."

子曰:"《关雎》乐而不淫，哀而不伤。"

——《论语》

3. Zixia asked, "what is the meaning of these lines: 'Her entrancing smile, dimpling, Her beautiful eyes so animated and clear. White renders the colors vibrant

and distinct'?" The Master said, "White is applied after the colors are put in."

子夏问曰："'巧笑倩兮，美目盼兮，素以为绚兮。'何谓也？"子曰："绘事后素。"

——《论语》

4. When the Master was singing with others and liked a particular song, he would invariably ask that the song be repeated before he should join in.

子与人歌而善，必使反之，而后和之。

——《论语》

5. The Master heard the *shao* music when he was in Qi. For the next three months, he did not notice the taste of meat. He said, "I never imagined that music could be this beautiful."

子在齐闻《韶》，三月不知肉味，曰："不图为乐之至于斯也。"

——《论语》

Part IV   Vocabulary Treasure

1. **hinge**   *v.*   attach with a hinge

   A good life **hinges** on diligence. With diligence, one does not have to fear about shortages.

   民生在勤，勤则不匮。

2. **nutrient**   *adj.*   of or providing nourishment

   The **nutrients** for a giant tree come from the root of the tree.

   树高千尺，营养在根。

3. **ideal**   *adj.*   conforming to an ultimate standard of perfection or excellence; embodying an ideal

   For the **ideal** that I hold dear to my heart, I will not regret a thousand depth to die.

亦余心之所向兮，虽九死其犹未悔。

4. **ensure**   *v.*   make certain of

It is only with reform that we can **ensure** continuous existence and growth.

如将不尽，与古为新。

5. **embark**   *v.*   proceed somewhere despite the risk of possible dangers

That is half of the people who have **embarked** on one hundred mile journey may fall by the wayside.

行百里者半九十。

6. **prosperity**   *n.*   an economic state of growth with rising profits and full employment

Embarking on a journey toward a higher goal of common **prosperity**, China is committed to providing a happy and dignified life for some one-fifth of the world's population.

中国正在朝着共同富裕的更高目标迈进，致力于让世界上约五分之一的人口过上幸福有尊严的生活。

7. **democracy**   *n.*   a system of government in which people choose their rulers by voting for them in elections

China's whole-process people's **democracy**, which is democracy in its broadest, most genuine and most effective form, is the defining feature of socialist democracy.

中国实行的全过程人民民主，是最广泛、最真实、最有效的民主，是社会主义民主的本质特征。

8. **sustained**   *adj.*   maintained at length without interruption or weakening

Despite facing challenges amid a cloudy global outlook, they said China has the solid foundation and conditions to achieve **sustained** growth with the support of its ultra-large domestic market and complete industrial chains, with the country having plenty of room for monetary easing and strong fiscal stimulus.

尽管面临全球前景不明朗的情况，但中国拥有庞大的国内市场和完整的产业链，有充足的空间放松货币政策和实施强有力的财政刺激，中国有实现持续增长的坚实基础和条件。

9. **masterpiece** *n.* the most outstanding work of a creative artist or craftsman

International Space Station are coming to a halt, after which this **masterpiece** of space cooperation is expected to be de-orbited by 2030.

国际空间站即将停运，这一太空合作的杰作预计将在 2030 年脱离轨道。

10. **aesthetic** *adj.* relating to the enjoyment or study of beauty, or showing great beauty

We will fully implement the Party's educational policy, carry out the basic task of fostering virtue through education, and nurture a new generation of capable young people with sound moral grounding, intellectual ability, physical vigor, **aesthetic** sensibility, and work skills who will fully develop socialism and carry forward the socialist cause.

全面贯彻党的教育方针，落实立德树人根本任务，培养德智体美劳全面发展的社会主义建设者和接班人。

Part V Language Practice

1. Translate the following paragraph into English.

爱德华·蒙克是挪威著名的表现主义画家。人们可以在他的画中看出，那些最坏的日子对于他来说如同一笔财富，他是用整个心灵来创作的。他根据自己亲身经历，通过主题来表现对生存和死亡的感受。每一幅画都强烈地传达着画家的感受和情绪。也许艺术的魅力就在于警示后人，疾病与死亡是任何人都无法摆脱的，学会直面病魔与死亡，直面人生，珍惜生命。

2. Critical Thinking

This part is to improve the critical thinking ability by writing a composition.

Direction: Write a composition on the topic: Art and Medicine. The composition is based on the following information, and it is at least 120 words.

> ➢ the common goal of art and medicine
> ➢ the differences between art and medicine
> ➢ my opinion

Part VI   Further Reading

1. Xanthelasma and Lipoma in Leonardo da Vinci's Mona Lisa

The Mona Lisa is a half-length portrait of a woman by the Italian artist Leonardo da Vinci. It has been acclaimed as the best known, the most visited, the most written about, the most parodied work of art in the world. Every year, millions of people queued in order to cast a glance at the Mona Lisa for 20 seconds or so. Mona Lisa is among the greatest attractions in the Louvre.

But we can enjoy this painting from a different perspective. Let's stand back and talk to Mona Lisa, just like a physician listening to the patient to discover the diagnosis. We can see skin alterations at the inner end of the left upper eyelid similar to xanthelasma, and a swelling of the dorsum of the right hand suggestive of a subcutaneous lipoma. These findings in a woman of 25—30 years old, who died at the age of 37, may be indicative of essential hyperlipidemia, a strong risk factor for ischemic heart disease in middle age. As far as is known, this portrait of Mona Lisa painted in 1506 is the first evidence that xanthelasma and lipoma were prevalent in the sixteenth century.

2. What are the symbols of cultural blending in thangka, 'Oriental Oil Painting'?

Thangka, once called "Oriental Oil Painting" in the West, has been passed down on Tibet's snowy plateau for more than 1,000 years. This art form, focuses on drawing scenes within square inches. Thangka is very close to Western oil painting in its processes, with its artistic forms and techniques influenced not only by Indian and Nepalese painting styles, but also deeply by Tang Dynasty painting styles and landscape painting in the Central Plains. Liu Yang, an associate professor in Tibet University's College of Art, recently gave China News Service's East-West Quest an exclusive interview.

China News Service: Why is thangka, which is full of mystery, widely sought-after by collectors?

Liu: Thangka is mysterious because people don't know enough about it. It is divided into hand-painted and non-hand-painted. Hand-painted thangka is actually a scroll painting with agate, coral, cinnabar and other natural precious minerals as pigments, painted on cloth curtains and framed with colored satin. The theme is mainly religion, involving history, politics, economy, culture, folklore, secular life and other fields, and thus thangka is called the "encyclopedia of Tibetan culture."

Traditional thangka integrates all of Tibetan culture, including history, landscape, culture, Tibetan medicine, astronomy, the calendar, etc. As a concrete embodiment of traditional skillful craftsmanship, it has high artistic appreciation value and collection value.

After thangka was selected for on China's National Intangible Cultural Heritage List in 2006, it was more sought-after by amateurs in China and abroad. In 2014, Liu Yiqian, a Chinese collector, bought an embroidered thangka of the Emperor Yongle in the Ming Dynasty for HKD 348 million ($44.3 million), a record for the auction amount of thangka so far, making this art form quickly become the focus of attention.

Thangka painting, one of the most distinctive types of Chinese painting, is also one of the most important and distinctive painting forms in Tibet. Today, people can see many thangka cultural relics with a history of thousands of years in the Potala Palace, the Tibet Museum or temples with their colors still bright and dazzling.

Why does thangka not fade easily? Thangka has a unique side in paintings all over the world: it is made from gold, silver and other precious stones, all of which come from natural minerals. In addition, the painter's color-matching ratio, coloring techniques and other techniques make its pigments very firm, and they don't fall off easily. In addition, the preservation method is also very important. People in Tibet think that offering thangka is very sacred, and they are very careful in keeping it. The scroll is easy to carry, which is very suitable for people in Tibet, who lived a nomadic life in ancient times. It is taken out and displayed on the special occasions only.

CNS: Westerners once called thangka "Oriental Oil Painting." What is the difference between its artistic expression and oil painting?

Liu: Thangka's form of expression and painting process are very close to oil painting. For example, before thangka painting, it is necessary to stretch, glue and polish the canvas. When making drafts, it is necessary to use charcoal strips or pencils to outline lines on canvas and color the back. Hence, some Westerners who have just come into contact with thangka called thangka "Oriental Oil Painting."

Thangka has different aesthetic characteristics from traditional Chinese painting and oil painting, with not only basic aesthetics of image modeling, but also symbolism and aestheticism.

CNS: How does thangka witness the history of the exchanges between Central Plains and Tibet. How do its painting elements interact with traditional Chinese painting to form its own characteristics?

Liu: In the history of Chinese civilization, all ethnic groups have made common progress and development through exchanges, communication and blending. The inheritance and development of thangka have absorbed the essence of all ethnic cultures.

Nowadays, thangka art instruction has also been introduced into middle-school art classes, which is a brand-new attempt and pioneering undertaking. It can enable students to encounter and understand traditional Tibetan art as soon as possible and broaden the thinking of artistic creation, thus playing a positive role in improving students' comprehensive artistic ability.

The integration of cultures has brought innovation and development. Innovating thangka is a challenge to every artist. Through bold imagination and a free combination of thangka elements, the new life and customs in Tibet are expressed by using various expressive skills of thangka painting and highly generalized artistic techniques, thus forming a unique artistic style in which truth, beauty and goodness are ubiquitous, which we call "new thangka".

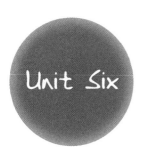

Unit Six

Art for Art's Sake

Part I Pre-Reading Task

A video clip of a choir comprising 36 geriatrics singing a popular song titled *Adolescents* during an online gala to celebrate Lunar New Year in early February went viral and inspired many younger viewers.

These seniors, who are age 75 on average, clad in dress shirts and bowties, won thunderous applause from the audience in the studio after their performance at the gala. Many Internet users have also expressed their admiration of the group's spirited display.

"I don't see their silver hair. I only see their ardent affection for life. It is because of such affection that they've been crowned by the brilliant radiance of time," reads a comment by a netizen with the username Sirlin.

The elderly singers, however, aren't just regular senior citizens with a penchant for music.

Formed in 2008, the choir is made up of more than 100 alumni of China's prestigious Tsinghua University. In fact, many of those who took to the stage for the gala show are regarded as the unsung heroes behind China's rapid development over the decades.

Questions:

1. Are you impressed after reading the news report?

2. Are you fond of singing? Can you sing this song for us?

3. Are you willing to invite your grandparents to sing this song together?

Part II   Reading Task

● Israeli artist Eyal Gever is working on a project that will be the first artwork created in space. It will be a 3D sculpture made inside the International Space Station. He will create his artwork using a zero-gravity 3D printer. Once it is finished, the sculpture will be released into the universe.

Working with NASA, Gever's space project is named "Laugh". The 3D printer will produce a physical representation of a person's laugh. Sound cannot travel in space, but this sculpture can show what laughter looks like.

Gever is asking people around the world to participate in his project. There is a social media campaign called "LaughInSpace", where people are invited to record and submit their laughter online. When the audio samples have been collected, people will be invited to vote on which clip should be represented in the sculpture. Then Gever will use the sounds of the winner's laughter to create the space sculpture.

Questions:

1. Can you describe an impressive sculpture that you have seen?

2. What do you think is the purpose of creating a piece of artwork in the outer space?

3. If you are allowed to send a piece of artwork into the universe, what are you going to send?

● Interviewer: Kathy Richards is a specialist art tour guide. Kathy, can you tell us what trends you've noticed in recent years?

Kathy: Well, one of the biggest phenomena I've noticed is a huge increase in visitors to galleries and a growing interest in modern art in general.

Interviewer: What do you think the reason is for that?

Kathy: Well, there are several reasons, I think. The most important ones are firstly, that some new contemporary art galleries have opened which have had a lot of publicity, and secondly the younger generation feel more comfortable with modern art so the kind of people visiting galleries is changing. Finally, the new generation of galleries have become destinations in themselves...they tend to be housed in amazing buildings...

Questions:

1. Are there any art galleries in your city? Do people in your city like visiting art museums and galleries?
2. Have you ever visited any art museums or galleries? What do you learn from these art galleries and museums?
3. Do you think it is beneficial for children to go to art museums and galleries?

● The National Art Museum of China (NAMOC) is the only national art museum of plastic arts in China. Starting to be built in 1958, NAMOC, with its title board inscribed by Chairman Mao Zedong, was formally open to the public in 1963. NAMOC is a national cultural landmark after foundation of the People's Republic of China.

NAMOC integrates exhibition, collection, research, public education, international exchange, restoration of artworks and cultural and creative industries. It is the highest hall of fine arts in China and also a public cultural service platform. The robust development of NAMOC benefits greatly from the support of the central government and the direct leadership of the Ministry of Culture. The government has established a special collection fund, which laid a solid foundation for the museum's collection of art treasure. Quite a few collectors and artists donated their collections to the country out of their social responsibility and strong belief in "art serving the people", which contributes to rich collections of NAMOC.

Since its establishment, NAMOC has held thousands of various influential exhibitions, which not only reflect development and prosperity of Chinese art but also provide an important platform of artistic exchange between China and the world. NAMOC shoulders the cultural responsibility of "promoting outstanding traditional culture, collecting all kinds of fine arts, strengthening international and domestic exchanges, facilitating contemporary artistic creation, building the peak of fine arts and benefiting public cultural services." Adhering to "Xi Jinping Thought on Socialism with Chinese Characteristics for a New Era", NAMOC will remain true to its original aspiration, keep its mission firmly in mind, and work tirelessly to realize the Chinese Dream of national rejuvenation.

Questions:

1. According to the article, what service can NAMOC provide?
2. Some people claim that art museums and art galleries will not be needed because people can see historical objects and works of art by using a computer. Do you agree or disagree with this opinion?
3. What role can art museums and art galleries play in realizing the Chinese Dream of national rejuvenation?

● Voice-over: *The Mona Lisa*, the most famous painting in the world, was truly revolutionary even in its time. While he was painting *the Mona Lisa*, Leonardo da Vinci broke all the rules, even his own. In spite of the fact that Leonardo and other artists believed that women should only be portrayed with eyes gazing slightly down, Leonardo painted *the Mona Lisa* looking directly at the viewer. The position of her body is another innovation. While her face looks straight ahead her body is slightly turned, a pose that creates a sense of movement and tension. In another break from tradition, *the Mona Lisa* is not wearing any jewelry or adornments. Finally, backgrounds in portraits usually indicated a real place but the landscape in Leonardo's portrait seems almost imaginary.

Questions:

1. According to the script, what makes *the Mona Lisa* so revolutionary?
2. In creating artwork, which one is more important, innovation or tradition?
3. What do you think can be done to balance innovation and tradition?

• Anne: When I was young, um, I was always interested in, um, reading books about people and, and the dynamics, different kinds of relationships they had and so when I became a painter it was natural for me to be interested in painting people and looking for similar kinds of stories to tell about them, that you might read about in a book.

Questions:

1. How can a painter's reading influence his or her artwork?
2. Do you like reading? How does reading change your life?
3. Do you know any painting that tells a story?

Part III   Moral Tips

1. The tools of art are images, colors, or sounds, which are not only not afraid of being destroyed by science, but are increasingly developed by science, and the tools of artistic expression have suddenly been very advanced.

艺术的表现工具是形象、颜色，或声音，这种东西不但不怕科学来摧残，乃以科学日见发达，反使艺术的表现工具得到迅猛提升。

——林风眠

2. Public art is an important carrier and symbol of a city's cultural spirit, aesthetic characteristics and citizens' cultural temperament. It should show its creative, public welfare and regional cultural values in terms of showing the aesthetic culture and humanistic spirit of the urban public environment, as well as in creating various public spaces and communication places in urban daily life, and serve the public life and cultural welfare of citizens. At the same time, public art is also an important driving force and way to enhance the cultural literacy of citizens and promote the cultural construction of urban communities themselves.

公共艺术是一座城市的文化精神、审美特征以及市民文化气质的重要载体和象征。它理应在显现城市公共环境的审美文化和人文精神方面，以及在营造城市日常生活中的各种公共空间及交往场所方面，显现其创造性、公益性和地域性的文化价值，为市民的公共生活和文化福利而服务。公共艺术同时也是提升市民文化素养和促进城市社区自身文化建设的重要推手和途径。

——翁剑青

3. Art should serve the public, and artists must first start from the actual needs of the people, understand the issues they care about and the ability to accept art.

艺术要服务于大众，艺术家首先要从人民大众的实际需要出发，要了解他们关心的问题和艺术接受的能力。

——邵大箴

4. In fact, literary and artistic innovation is not only the update of technology, but also the docking of writers and artists' minds and creativity. "Our journey is the sea of stars", only by holding this kind of mind and feeling can the artist "cage the heaven and the earth in the form, and frustrate all things in the pen", and dedicate good works with unlimited creativity.

事实上，文艺创新既是技术的更新，更是作家艺术家胸怀和创意的对接。"我们的征途是星辰大海"，艺术家只有抱定这种胸怀和情怀，才能"笼天地于形内，挫万物于笔端"，奉献出创意无限的好作品。

——张江

5. A life, a picture, a picture, everyone encounters, due to the difference in status, feeling emotions, is different. However, this period of life, if it is described in a novel, played in music, this nature, if it is painted on the picture album and sung in love words, it will surely attract the attention and empathy of the whole society.

一段人生，一幅自然，各人遇之，因地位关系之差别，感觉情绪，毫不相同。但是这一段人生，若是描写小说之中，弹奏于音乐之里，这一幅自然，若是绘画于图册之上，歌咏于情词之中，则必引起全社会的注意与同感。

——宗白华

Part IV   Vocabulary Treasure

1. **contemporary**   *adj.*   belong to the present time
With lights fading out at the Neilson Studio of Sydney Dance Company, 18-year-old Australian **contemporary** dancer Xanthe, together with dozens of her peers, quietly walked on the center stage, ready to showcase the fruits of their Chinese martial arts training.
悉尼舞蹈团尼尔森工作室的灯光渐渐熄灭，18 岁的澳大利亚当代舞者桑特和她的几十名同龄人一起，静静地走在舞台中央，准备展示他们的中国武术训练的成果。

2. **revolutionary**   *adj.*   involving a great or complete change
China's Shanghai on Thursday announced the first batch of its **revolutionary** cultural relics of over 350 buildings and artifacts, as the Communist Party of China (CPC) celebrates its centenary this year.
在今年中国共产党庆祝成立一百周年之际，上海市第一批革命文物名录于周四公布，其中包括三百五十多处建筑物和文物。

3. **innovative**   *adj.*   introducing or using new ideas, ways of doing sth,

etc.

Despite China's efforts to develop vocational training, it is still not that attractive and there exist many obstacles to improving the quality of industrial workers and cultivating more "outstanding craftsmen". More **innovative** practices are needed and the existing social evaluation system still has room for improvement.

尽管中国为发展职业培训做出了努力，但吸引力仍然不大，提高行业工人的素质和培养更多"杰出工匠"仍然存在许多障碍。我们仍需要更多的创新做法，并且现有的社会评价体系仍有改进的空间。

4. **imaginary** *adj.* existing only in your mind or imagination

A recently published children's science book series, *The Natural History in the Palace Museum*, collects images of these real and **imaginary** creatures that once mesmerized Emperor Qianlong.

最近出版的儿童科普丛书《故宫博物馆里的自然史》收集了那些曾经令乾隆着迷的真实的和虚构的生物图像。

5. **dynamics** *n.* the forces or properties which stimulate growth, development, or change within a system or process

A sector-by-sector breakdown of the NBS figures reveals improved economic structure and new **dynamics** in emerging industries.

对国家统计局数据逐个部门细分，揭示了新兴产业经济结构的改善和新的动力。

Part V Language Practice

1. Translate the following paragraph into Chinese.

Beijing Opera is the cream of the Chinese culture. As a traditional art form, its costumes and facial masks are more popular with people. Different styles of costumes are used to reflect the status of different characters. There are more decorations in the costumes of nobles, while those of the poor tend to be simple and less elemental. Facial masks can reflect qualities of different characters. Facial masks using different colors are important ways to portray a character. People can tell a hero from a villain by the colors of the masks. In general, white usually represents treachery, black righteousness, yellow bravery, and blue and green rebellious fighters, while gold and silver divinity and Buddhism.

2. Critical Thinking

This part is to improve the critical thinking ability by writing a composition.

Direction: Write a composition on the topic: Do you think art plays an important role in our life? The composition is based on the following information, and it is at least 120 words.

> ➢ **art's role in our life**
>
> ➢ **examples**
>
> ➢ **my opinion**

Part VI   Further Reading

1. Craftsman turns reeds into creative,
valuable art works

For many, reeds are nothing but grass, but in Wei Lichu's hands, they are turned into art.

Wei, 55, is a fine arts teacher at a vocational school in Lindian county, Northeast China's Heilongjiang province. Using an electric soldering iron and dye, he creates images on various kinds of reeds.

Ahead of the Year of the Ox, that started on Feb 12, he completed a 1.66-meter-long piece based on the traditional Chinese painting, Five Oxen. "It took me over 20 days using various kinds of reeds and techniques," says

Wei.

In Wei's hometown, reeds grow everywhere in wetlands and the wilderness. When he was young, his family often used reeds, measuring more than two meters, to make mats.

In 1992, Wei started focusing on reed handicrafts and established a studio the following year.

China has a reed-handicraft history stretching back hundreds of years. In 2013, the craft was listed into the provincial-level intangible cultural heritage.

Each reed harvest season, Wei buys a whole truck of reeds.

"We can only use 250 kilograms out of a load weighing a metric ton, and all must be selected manually," says Wei.

Stiff reeds are difficult to iron and paint, he says, while those that are too soft will break easily. Reed handicraft involves multiple steps. First, one side of a reed needs to be cut with a knife. It is then flattened, soaked in warm water, and ironed. The ironing time determines the color of the raw materials.

Dyeing the reeds requires special weak alkaline pigments, which need to be accurately boiled.

"Even a minute's difference in boiling time will lead to the wrong color," Wei says.

Some 300 of his works, including animals, flowers and figures, have been sold to more than 10 countries including Russia, Japan and Sweden. The most expensive work, which is decorated with cranes and measures 24 meters in length, was sold at a price of 400,000 yuan ($62,000).

"Art is interlinked and can become a bridge of friendship. Although cultural backgrounds are different, many foreigners can understand the content expressed in the artworks," Wei says.

Recently, Wei has been producing reed artworks themed on *Water Margin*, one of the four classical novels in Chinese literature.

"I hope to spread more traditional Chinese culture through reed crafts so that more people can feel the beauty in it," he says.

2. Arts even more key after poverty victory

Literature and arts can play an even more important role as China has clinched victory in eradicating absolute poverty and entered the stage of rural vitalization, said Fan Di'an, member of the CPPCC National Committee, at an interview on Thursday afternoon at the Great Hall of the People in Beijing.

"Chinese literature and arts have the tradition of building up the spiritual value and meaning of life, and excellent artworks play an important role in boosting mental strength," said Fan, who is also chairman of the China Artists Association and dean of the Central Academy of Fine Arts.

Fan said that in the past years, writers and artists have visited many impoverished places to witness poverty alleviation efforts, inspiring them to produce an abundance of works of literature and art.

"Those works have resonated with audiences, and people love works which depict the reality of people's lives, tell the truth and reveal true feelings," he said.

"On the other hand, we need to tell more stories about millions of poverty relief cadres and hundreds of millions of Chinese farmers," Fan told the media before sitting at the opening ceremony of the fourth session of the 13th National Committee of the Chinese People's Political Consultative Conference.

He said that writers and artists can participate in the construction of rural civilization by studying local culture and protecting village's history, especially the precious ancient dwellings and culture.

"The villages are rich in traditional ethnic handicrafts and intangible cultural heritage, which need to be enlivened to facilitate the revitalization of rural cultural industries," he said.

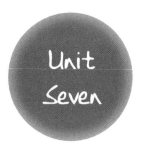

Unit Seven

Beauty of Art Learning

Part I   Pre-Reading Task

While few people would associate inanimate objects such robots with having artistic capabilities, the ongoing 2017 World Robot Conference in Beijing is shedding light on their creative abilities.

Wearing a peaked cap and glasses, and sporting a handlebar mustache, the 1.55-meter-tall artist robot stands in silence, fully devoting to sketching portraits of visitors in black ink.

Saidaqian was created by Shenzhen Academy of Robotics. A user's photo can be sent to the robot's system, it will then begin to draw the portrait, taking around five minutes to complete it.

According to Fang Siwen from the academy, Saidaqian's appearance was designed to resemble the stereotype of foreign street artists. The robot can be used in museums, shopping malls and restaurants to teach drawing or attract customers.

The company has already sold two portrait robots prior to the conference, at a price of around 300,000 yuan ($45,000) each. Customers can also rent a robot for nearly 8,000 yuan per month, said Fang.

Questions:

1. Do you want Saidaqian to draw a portrait for you?

2. Do you like drawing with pencils, or using computers? Why?

3. Did you take any painting classes when you were a little kid? Did you like having painting classes? Why?

Part II   Reading Task

● For a month in the spring of 1987, my wife Ellen and I lived in the bustling eastern Chinese city of Nanjing with our 18-month-old son Benjamin while studying arts education in Chinese kindergartens and elementary schools.

I soon realized that this incident was directly relevant to our assigned tasks in China: to investigate the ways of early childhood education (especially in the arts), and to throw light on Chinese attitudes toward creativity.

Questions:

Describe an art course that you have attended.

1. What was the course? What did you do in the course?

2. Was it useful? Why?

3. In the course, which part was the most difficult for you? And how did you deal with that?

● Children as young as 5 or 6 were painting flowers, fish and animals with the skill and confidence of an adult; calligraphers 9 and 10 years old were producing works that could have been displayed in a museum.

Questions:

1. Do you usually write with a writing brush?

2. What is calligraphy? What are the Four Treasures of the Study?

3. Someone argues that computers might one day replace handwriting. Is it necessary for us to practice our handwriting with writing brushes?

● The idea that learning should take place by continual careful shaping and molding applies equally to the arts. Watching children at work in a classroom setting, we were astonished by their facility. In a visit to the homes of two of the young artists, we learned from their parents that they worked on perfecting their craft for several hours a day.

Questions:

Describe an art teacher who has greatly influenced you in your life.

1. What subject did he/she teach?

2. What was special about him/her?

3. In what ways were you influenced by him/her?

Part III   Moral Tips

1. As a renowned Chinese artist well exposed to the Western education, Liu Haisu pioneered both the fine arts movement and modern art education in China. He was highly recognized as a scholar "fully dedicating himself to art, education and innovation". For all his altruistic pursuits, he donated all his valuable art works and collections of painting and calligraphy works from various Chinese dynasties to the country in his old age. Liu Haisu Art Museum, based on Liu Haisu's generous donation, in a sense, purportedly showcases and disseminates Liu Haisu's unceasing endeavors in art and education.

刘海粟先生学贯中西，是中国著名的艺术家，更是中国新美术运动的拓荒者和现代美术教育的奠基人。他一生追求艺术，一生致力于美术教育事业，一生艰苦创新。晚年，他将自己毕生创作的主要作品和收藏的历代书画作品全部无偿捐献给国家。刘海粟美术馆以刘海粟先生的丰厚捐赠为根基，将刘海粟先生开辟的艺术道路和追求的美育理想加以传承和发扬光大。

2. Chinese calligraphy (shu fa) refers to writing art and techniques with writing brushes. 1,600 years ago, a boy named Wang Xizhi worked hard at calligraphy. He washed his writing brushes in a pool and the pool turned black. Eventually he became a prominent calligrapher in China. Writing brushes, Chinese inks, rice paper and ink slabs are the basic tools of calligraphy. Proper technique for handling the writing brushes and maintaining the proper angle between the tips of brushes and the paper are required. The structure of each individual character and overall arrangement are both important. Calligraphers have created plenty of masterpieces which have been passed from generation to generation. One of the masterpieces is the *Orchid Pavilion Preface* by Wang Xizhi. Shu Fa represents the aesthetic taste and philosophy of Chinese scholars.

中国书法通常是指用毛笔书写的艺术和技法。1600多年前的王羲之勤练书法。他刷洗毛笔的墨汁把池塘都染成了黑色，后来他成为中国最受尊崇的书法家。笔、墨、纸、砚是书法的基本工具。书法，讲求握笔的姿势，注意笔尖和纸的角度。也讲究单个字的结构和整体的布局。几千年里，书法家们创作了诸多传世名作。王羲之的《兰亭集序》便是其中之一。可以说书法蕴含着中国文人的审美情趣和人生哲学。

3. Born in 1982, Lang Lang, a famous Chinese concert pianist, started playing the piano when he was three. According to him, he was inspired by the episode *The Cat Concerto* in *Tom and Jerry*. From then on, he practiced the piano every day. When he was nine, Lang moved to Beijing with his father, who quit his job. And he worked even harder. After six years of hard work and struggling together with his father in Beijing, he won major competitions including the Xinghai National Piano Competition in 1993 as well as first prize for outstanding artistic performance at the 4th International Competition for Young Pianists in Ettlingen, Germany in 1994. In 1997, at 15 years of age, Lang began further

studies at the Curtis Institute of Music in Philadelphia.

Lang's professional career officially began in 1998. He has performed all over the world on average 120 times a year. In 2008, the young pianist established the Lang Lang International Music Foundation and started the "Keys of Inspiration" music class program in 2013 with the objective of igniting children's passion for music. Lang believes that every kid has the right to learn music.

郎朗，中国著名钢琴演奏家，出生于 1982 年，三岁时开始弹奏钢琴。他提到，《猫和老鼠》这部动画片中的《猫的协奏曲》这集激励着他。从那时起，他每天练习钢琴。九岁的时候，郎朗和父亲一起搬到了北京，父亲辞掉了工作。他也更加努力了。郎朗在北京与父亲共同奋斗了六年。在此期间，他赢得了许多重要比赛，包括 1993 年星海杯全国钢琴比赛。1994 年郎朗在德国埃特林根举行的第四届国际青少年钢琴家比赛中获得杰出艺术表现一等奖。1997 年，15 岁的郎朗开始在费城柯蒂斯音乐学院深造。

郎朗的职业生涯正式开始于 1998 年。他平均每年在世界各地演出 120 次。2008 年，这位年轻的钢琴家成立了郎朗国际音乐基金会，并于 2013 年启动了"琴键与灵感"音乐课程，旨在点燃孩子们对音乐的热情。郎朗相信每个孩子都有学习音乐的权利。

Part IV   Vocabulary Treasure

1. **desirable**   *adj.*   you would like to have or do; worth having or doing
   "The ETS, as it is currently designed, will have a very marginal impact on reducing emissions," said Li Shuo, a policy adviser at Greenpeace China. "A cap-and-trade system without absolute emissions-based trading benchmarks is a convoluted exercise." Li also said it would be **desirable** for Beijing to set a five-year 2021—2025 timeline for action to tackle climate change, possibly unveiled later this year.
   绿色和平中国政策顾问李硕表示："按照目前的设计，碳排放交易系统对减排的影响非常小。"没有基于绝对排放量的交易基准的总量管制与排放交易制度是一项复杂的工作。"李硕还表示，北京制定一个（2021—2025 年）为期五年的应对气候变化的时间表是可取的，计划表可能会在今年晚些时候公布。

2. **in due course**　when it is the right time

China will also promote the optimization and structural adjustment of State-owned capital and focus on strategic emerging industries to form new central SOE groups **in due course**, to deepen the country's supply-side structural reform and support innovation-based growth, Hao said.

郝鹏表示，中国还将推动国有资本优化结构调整，适时以战略性新兴产业为重点组建新的中央国有企业集团，深化供给侧结构性改革，支持创新型增长。

3. **misdeed**　*n.*　a wrong or wicked act

Almost every year, there are brands that get into this trouble out of carelessness or intended moves. They have all paid a heavy price for that **misdeed**, and the price they pay is a good reminder never to repeat that folly again.

几乎每年都有品牌因为粗心或有意的举动而陷入这样的麻烦。他们都为这一罪行付出了沉重的代价，他们付出的代价是一个很好的提醒，永远不再重复这种蠢事。

4. **priority**　*n.*　sth. that one must do before anything else; sth. that holds a high place among competing claims

While the **priority** is reducing tutoring and homework, the other is improving schools' provision of activities and sports. "If quality programs can be delivered in schools, supported by increased spending from the government on the public education system, then there is no doubt that the education system will be better and more equitable," he said.

第一要务是减少家教和家庭作业，第二要务是改善学校提供的活动和运动项目。他说："如果学校能够提供高质量的项目，并得到政府对公共教育系统增加支出的支持，那么毫无疑问，教育系统将更好、更公平。"

5. **self-reliance**   *n.*   able to do or decide things by yourself, rather than depending on other people for help

While addressing the general assemblies of the members of the Chinese Academy of Sciences and the Chinese Academy of Engineering in late May, President Xi Jinping, also general secretary of the Communist Party of China Central Committee and chairman of the Central Military Commission, called for accelerated efforts in building China into a leader in science and technology and achieving more **self-reliance** in science and technology.

在5月下旬向中国科学院、中国工程院院士大会致辞时，中共中央总书记、中央军委主席、国家主席习近平要求加快建设科技强国，增强科技自主能力。

Part V   Language Practice

1. Translate the following paragraph into Chinese.

Longmen Grottoes are located in the south of Luoyang city. Longmen Grottoes, Yungang Caves and Mogao Caves are regarded as three most famous grottoes in China. Lots of historical materials concerning art, music, religion, calligraphy, medicine, costume and architecture are kept in Longmen Grottoes. There are as many as 100,000 statues within the 1,400 caves, ranging from 1 inch to 57 feet in height. These works that are entirely devoted to the Buddhist religion represent the peak of Chinese stone carving art.

2. Critical Thinking

This part is to improve the critical thinking ability by writing a composition.

Directions: Write a composition on the topic: What benefits can you get from art classes? The composition is based on the following information, and it is at least 120 words.

> ➢ **to think creatively**
> ➢ **to develop oneself physically and mentally**
> ➢ **my opinion**

Part VI   Further Reading

1. How should we guide children in art?

An interactive art session for children was held last weekend in the famed scenic water town of Wuzhen, east China's Zhejiang province, to encourage children's talent in creating hand-made art pieces.

Themed "The Future Creature," the two-day art session motivated children to think about the definition of life, and what will the planet's creatures, especially humans, be like in the far future. Around 40 families participated in the activity.

Huang Lin, a modern artist and teacher in China, hosted the event. During the class he explored the possibilities of future creatures with the children and showed them how to combine various materials like paper, wooden chips, magazine pages, and straws by applying skills like painting, cutting, and pasting.

The children and their parents were left to create their own work in a free way.

The art without boundaries

According to Jiang Yijing, a 10-year-old girl who participated in the activity, the event was quite different from the art class at school where the art textbook often set some requirements for the pupils, and art teachers also evaluate the artwork according to those standards.

"I can create whatever I want today," Jiang said.

Art education among children: What's next?

According to Sohu, more than 79 percent of the parents would sign up for extracurricular classes, art classes or supplementary learning courses for their kids during the summer vacation. According to a survey by *People's Daily* in Guangzhou, more than 60 percent of the local parents have signed up for extracurricular classes for their children at weekends.

Some families have a healthy ecology in choosing those art classes, by respecting the children's interests, while many others revealed their anxiety about their kids' competitiveness. "Don't want the children to lose at the starting line" was the most frequently mentioned quote during the survey.

In this context, the goal of art education gets blurred. Why should children get access to art, and learn to create art at an early age?

"What is the essence of art?" Huang said, "It's opening our hearts and giving everyone more freedom and their own way of expression." His point of view may pose a better reason for children to learn art in the future.

2. History of Central Academy of Fine Arts

The Central Academy of Fine Arts was originally the National Art School in Beiping. The history of National Art School in Beiping might date back to the founding of the National School of Fine Arts in Beijing in 1918, advocated by the notable educator, Cai Yuanpei. Zheng Jin, a famous art educator, served as the first principal of the National School of Fine Arts in Beijing. It was the first national school of fine arts in Chinese history, and also the beginning of Chinese modern education of fine arts.

In November 1949, the National Art School in Beiping merged with the department of fine arts at third campus of North China University, which was originally the department of fine arts at Luxun Academy of Arts in Yan'an founded in 1938. Authorized by the Central People's Government, the National School of Fine Arts was founded. Chairman Mao Zedong wrote the school's name. Xu Beihong served as the first president.

In January 1950, approved by the Government Administration Council of the Central People's Government, it was officially named the Central Academy of Fine Arts.

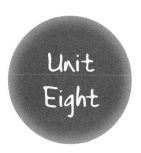

Unit Eight

Human Care in Health Care

Part I   Pre-Reading Task

The mission of AHHM (arts and humanities in health and medicine) is to engender a balance of science and humanities in order to foster the development of well-rounded health professionals who are skilled, caring and compassionate practitioners.

Life can be hard, and relationships are often difficult. In an era of fast advancing medical technology and rapidly changing medical ethics, a good physician-patient relationship is critically important for effective health care delivery. It may be reassuring to learn that the first steps in creating a trustworthy and positive physician-patient relationship are quite easy, which involve simple human courtesy and earnest communication, and the result can be mutual respect, knowledge and shared perspectives that improve the delivery of care:

1) treat the patient with respect

2) show empathy

3) practice good listening and make eye contact

4) ask the patient about themselves

5) explore the details of patient perspective about themselves

6) share the diagnosis clearly

7) engage the patient in setting the care plan

8) always pursue two-way conversations with the patient

Questions:

1. What is the mission of "arts and humanities in health and medicine"?

2. In order to become a good health care provider, what qualities of medical humanities should be developed?

3. In your opinion, what are good ways to create a good physician-patient relationship?

Part II   Reading Task

● Whether your role is that of a doctor or a health care administrator, working in the field of health care is both highly rewarding and challenging. Many medical procedures and treatments have both merits and downsides, and patients have their own input and circumstances to consider. The four principles of **health care ethics** provide **medical practitioners** with guidelines to make decisions when they inevitably face complicated situations involving patients. The four principles of health care ethics are autonomy, beneficence, non-maleficence and justice.

Questions:

1. What are the roles of a doctor or a health care administrator?

2. How to ensure patients are safe when being faced with some complicated medical situations?

3. What are the purposes of four principles of health care ethics, i.e. autonomy, beneficence, non-maleficence, and justice?

● **Autonomy**   In medicine, autonomy refers to the right of the patient to retain control over his or her body. A health care professional can suggest or advise, but any actions that attempt to persuade or coerce the patient into making a choice are violations of this principle. The patient must be allowed to make his or her own decisions—whether or not the medical service provider believes these choices are in that patient's best interests—independently and according to his or her personal values and beliefs.

Questions:

1. How do you understand autonomy, the first principle of health care ethics?
2. Do you agree that patients have their own rights to make clinical decisions? Why or why not?
3. Why is it important to allow patients to make independent decisions about treatment?

• **Beneficence**   This principle states that health care providers must do all they can to benefit the patient in each situation. All procedures and treatments recommended must be with the intention to do the most good for the patient. To ensure beneficence, medical practitioners must develop and maintain a high level of skill and knowledge, make sure that they are trained in the most current and best medical practices, and must consider their patients' individual circumstances, since what is good for one patient will not necessarily benefit another.

Questions:

1. What does the principle of beneficence refer to?
2. What must medical practitioners do in order to ensure beneficence?
3. What is the purpose of beneficence?

• **Non-Maleficence**   Non-maleficence is probably the best known of the four principles. In short, it means "to do no harm." This principle is intended to be the end goal for all of a practitioner's decisions, and it means that health care providers must consider whether other people or society could be harmed by a decision made, even if it is made for the benefit of an individual patient.

Questions:

1. What does non-maleficence mean in short?

2. Why is the principle of non-maleficence intended to be the end goal for all of a practitioner's decisions?

3. How to ensure the realization of the principle of non-maleficence in clinical practice?

● **Justice**　The principle of justice states that there should be an element of fairness in all medical decisions: fairness in decisions that burden and benefit, as well as equal distribution of scarce resources and new treatments. It advocates medical practitioners to uphold applicable laws and legislation when making choices.

Questions:

1. How do you understand justice, the fourth principle of health care ethics?

2. What examples can you give to illustrate the principle of justice?

3. What considerations should be taken in order to realize fairness in medical decisions?

Part III　Moral Tips

1. The expression "basic ethical principles" refer to those general judgements that serve as a basic justification for the many particular ethical prescriptions and evaluations of human actions.

"基本伦理原则"指在对特定的伦理规定、人类行为进行评判正当与否时所形成的一般判断。

2. In medicine, autonomy refers to the right of the patient to retain control over his or her body.

在医学上，"自主原则"指患者自己保留对其身体进行掌控的权利。

3. The principle of beneficence states that health care providers must do all they can to benefit the patient in each situation.

"有利原则"指出，医护人员必须在各种情况下尽其所能使患者受益。

4. In short, non maleficence means "to do no harm."

简而言之，"不伤害原则"的意思是"不给患者造成伤害"。

5. A doctor-patient relationship is a complex relationship between a doctor and a patient, which is built on trust, respect, communication and a common understanding of both the doctor and patients' sides.

医患关系是医生和患者之间的一种复杂关系，这种关系建立在医患双方彼此信任、相互尊重、有效沟通以及互相理解的基础之上。

Part IV   Vocabulary Treasure

1. **medical practitioner**   someone who practices medicine

Licensed **medical practitioner** in the context of health care means an individual other than a physician who is licensed or otherwise authorized by the state to provide health care services.

执业医师是指在医疗行业除医生以外的个人，他们有医师执照或经国家授权向他人提供医疗和健康照护服务。

2. compassionate *adj.* feeling or showing sympathy for people who are suffering

The challenges facing health care organizations are numerous and may change, but the primary goal remains steadfast: providing high-quality and **compassionate** health care for patients.

医疗机构正面临着众多挑战，这些挑战或许千变万化，但医疗机构的首要目标不曾改变：为患者提供高质量、富有同情心的医疗服务。

3. empathetic *adj.* able to understand how someone feels because you can imagine what it is like to be them

It may be that doctors, through their **empathetic** treatment, cause their patients to better manage their diabetes, or it may be that patients who do better managing their diabetes cause their doctors to think of themselves as more understanding, more involved, more empathetic.

医生通过共情治疗，或许可以帮助患者更好地进行糖尿病管理；而糖尿病管理较好的患者也可以让医生感受到，他们更善解人意、更关心、更具同理心。

4. sympathetic *adj.* kind to someone who has a problem and willing to understand how they feel

Empathetic and **sympathetic** are similar words, but they're not the same. While being empathetic means putting yourself completely in another person's shoes, being sympathetic means showing concern for someone when something bad happens to them.

共情和同情是两个相似词，但含义不同。共情意味着感同身受，能够站在他人立场上看待问题；而同情则意味着对他人发生的不幸表达怜悯之情。

5. health care the preservation of mental and physical health by preventing or treating illness through services offered by the health profession

The fundamental purpose of **health care** is to enhance quality of life by enhancing health. Commercial businesses focus on creating financial profit to support their valuation and remain viable. Health care must focus on creating social profit to fulfill its promise to society.

健康照护的根本目的在于通过提升健康水平进而提高生活质量。商业企业往往专注于创造利润以维持商业价值，保持商业活力，而医疗照护则必须注重创造社会价值，以履行其社会责任承诺。

6. **palliative care**   an interdisciplinary medical caregiving approach aimed at optimizing quality of life and mitigating suffering among people with serious, complex illness

Palliative care improves the quality of life of patients and that of their families who are facing challenges associated with life-threatening illness, whether physical, psychological, social or spiritual.

由于罹患危及生命的疾病，患者及其家人不得不面对来自身体、心理、社会或者精神层面的种种挑战，姑息疗法则可以改善他们的生活质量。

Part V   Language Practice

1. Translate the following principles of health care ethics into Chinese.

Autonomy   Beneficence   Non-maleficence   Justice

2. Critical Thinking

This part is to improve the critical thinking ability by writing a composition.

Direction: Write a composition on the topic: How to promote the relationship between doctors and patients? The composition is based on the following information, and it is at least 120 words.

  ➢ **treat the patient with respect**
  ➢ **show empathy**

➢ **practice good communication skills**

Part VI   Further Reading

Medical humanities play an important role in improving the doctor-patient relationship

The doctor-patient relationship is a complex social relationship that is affected by numerous factors. Three such factors are a lack of humanity in medicine, the predominance of techniques and technologies, and inappropriate administration of hospitals. All three of these problems are related to the absence of medical humanities. Hence, most efficient way to improve the doctor-patient relationship is to change the emphasis on medical science and to reshape medical humanities.

First, improve medical education by enhancing humanity. The key to resolving the tension between doctors and patients is reshaping the humanity of medical personnel. Improving medical humanities education is key to reshaping the humanity of doctors. There are inadequacies with medical humanities education in China. According to a survey, 88.7% of medical students indicated that their medical college does not have a framework for medical humanities education. In addition, medical education emphasizes knowledge about diseases, anatomy, and other technical subjects, and medical humanities courses account for only 8% of all medical courses.

Therefore, steps can be taken to enhance medical humanities in different stages of education. Medical colleges should expand their offerings in the humanities and increase the resources they devote to medical humanities education. Medical humanities must be promoted in conjunction with clinical training. Medical education should be problem-oriented and combined with clinical case studies. Simulated cases and role-playing are suited to medical humanities education and have gradually increased the level of thinking and behavior by medical students.

Medical humanities can be promoted in several ways during on-the-job training. Fostering humanity in medicine is a long-term process, and medical personnel can play a significant role in advocating humanity. Colleagues can learn from and compete with one another, thus enhancing their clinical skills and humanity. In addition, medical associations can advocate humanity among medical personnel and establish a standard for humane practices.

Second, end the predominance of techniques and technologies and bring back humanity to medicine. Medicine is a combination of natural science and human science in which both are essential. Medical development needs to find a proper balance between technology and humanity, and this requires the joint efforts of all sectors of society. Medicine itself must return to its origins, and medical ethics must be actively promoted to end "the predominance of techniques and technologies". The Doctor-Patient Relationship Course at the University of Chicago examine topics related to the doctor-patient relationship, communication between doctors and patients, and societal issues related to health. This course places medicine in a broader context in order to end "the predominance of technology" and to heighten awareness that technical and professional development are not the only parts of medicine.

Public discussions are also important since they affect how people view the human side of medicine. In China, the country's most largely read medical newspaper Health News, runs a special column on the human side of medicine. On television, medical documentaries such as "Life Matters" and "The Story in ER" present various aspects of the human side of medicine, helping the public to look at medicine from a fresh perspective. The media also has substantial ability to shape public opinion about doctors by dispelling the image of a doctor as an "angel" and instead providing the public with a more comprehensive view and by explaining the limitations of modern medicine since "medicine is not a panacea".

Third, provide humane administration to improve the patient experience. According to one study, only 20% of doctor-patient disputes are caused by medical technology. Medical equipment has become a greater part of the diagnostic process than communication. The patient experience is greatly affected by physical conditions, administrative procedures, and the medical procedure the patient is undergoing. Therefore, humanity needs to be fostered in hospital administration.

The internal administration of a hospital should focus on the "patient" and a method of assessment should be established to indicate the subjective quality of care. During treatment, the patient's views should be heeded and the patient's needs should be incorporated in hospital administration. A hospital should also enhance the humanity of medical personnel since their attitudes and mood will affect the relationship between doctors and patients. As an example, an employee assistance program (EAP) should be incorporated in hospital administration to help hospital employees address personal problems. Attending to the psychological and emotional needs of staff will help to resolve issues with the quality and efficiency of their work, reduce complaints and negative emotions, enhance the effectiveness of communication, and lead to a harmonious relationship.

Efforts have been made to improve the humane side of medicine and the relationship between doctors and patients, and these efforts should have a positive effect in the future.

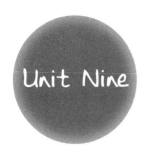

Unit Nine

Truth Exploration

Part I Pre-Reading Task

A 100-gram sample of lunar soil was added to the collection of the National Museum of China on Saturday and unveiled for public viewing.

It was among nearly 2 kilograms of lunar samples retrieved by China's Chang'e 5 mission late last year.

Chang'e 5, launched from the Wenchang Space Launch Center in Hainan province on Nov 24, touched down on the moon on Dec 1. The 23-day mission, which brought back lunar rocks and soil, was China's first such space endeavor.

The lunar soil is on display inside a specially designed transparent container at the museum. The synthetic quartz vessel replicates a zun, a bronze wine holder often used at rituals in the Shang (c.16th century—11th century BC) and Western Zhou (c.11th century—771 BC) dynasties.

The container is 38.44 centimeters tall, representing the average distance from the Earth to the Moon of 384,400 kilometers. The soil fills a globe, symbolizing the Moon, in the center of the container, which has a map of China at the base.

The sample is at the heart of an exhibition on the National Museum's ground floor that opened on Saturday and charts China's progress in space missions, especially lunar exploration.

In addition to the soil, the exhibition features dozens of objects, photos, videos and publications.

Highlights include the return capsule and parachute of the Chang'e 5 probe, as well as life-size models of its ascender and lander.

A model of the rover to be deployed by China's first Mars mission, Tianwen 1, is also being shown.

Wang Chunfa, the director of the National Museum, said at the opening of the exhibition that the museum has paid great attention to building a collection of objects showing China's major breakthroughs in science and displaying them.

He said the exhibition was mounted to celebrate this year's centenary of the founding of the Communist Party of China.

"The exhibition is to ignite people's interest in science...and to inspire people to dream, create and strive for the Chinese Dream of national rejuvenation," Wang said.

The museum has assembled dozens of objects related to China's space adventures, including the spacesuit worn by Yang Liwei, China's first astronaut.

It also has a long-term online exhibition—Dongfanghong Forever—that charts China's progress in aerospace technology in the past half century.

Bian Fangyue, a student at Beijing No.4 High School, was among the first members of the public to view the lunar soil.

"Chang'e 5 is a project of sophistication, and retrieving lunar soil marks a great leap in our nation's scientific development," he said. "I feel honored to be living in an era that has witnessed an achievement like this."

The National Museum has not said when the exhibition will end, but Wang said it will tour the country in the future.

Questions:

1. Why was the lunar soil displayed inside a bronze wine holder in the Shang and Western Zhou dynasties? What is the symbolic meaning?

2. What other objects were shown in this exhibition? What was the focus of this exhibition?

3. What is the great significance of this exhibition?

Part II   Reading Task

• Science is a fascinating exploration and investigation of discoveries that affect our daily lives. Science tries to understand the truth of the world. The knowledge generated by science is powerful and can be used to develop new technologies, treat diseases, and solve practical problems. A tiny discovery in science can transform the world and our lives greatly. For example, Sir Isaac Newton was inspired to formulate his theory of gravitation by watching an apple falling from a tree. This discovery changed the way people viewed the world around them. Millions of scientists all over the world are working to solve different parts of the puzzle of how the universe works. They are motivated by the thrill of understanding something that would otherwise remain a mystery. This is also true of the scientific thinkers of the past. Without their discoveries and inventions, today's modern world would not be modern at all. If you look back in history, all the great civilizations of the ancient world would have been contributed in some way to the advancement of science and technology.

Questions:

1. How do you understand the phrase "the truth of the world"?
2. Could you give an example of how "a tiny discovery in science can transform the world and our lives greatly"?
3. How to paraphrase the phrase "different parts of the puzzle of how the universe works"?

• The Scientific Revolution began in Europe in the 16th century and opened the door to modern science. Much of the work done in this period is considered the foundation of major fields of science, including physics, chemistry, biology and astronomy. The Scientific Revolution left the world with a more logical description of physics, in which the laws of motion and gravity were understood, setting the stage for many future breakthroughs and inventions, such as steam engines and rockets. In the field of biology, thinkers of the Scientific Revolution explained the physiology of the human body in terms of its mechanical properties, and paved the way for the advancement of illness prevention and treatment. With a better understanding of physics and mathematics, astronomers accepted the concept that the planets revolve around the sun.

Questions:

1. Try to find some information about the Scientific Revolution in the 16th century.
2. What are the "future breakthroughs and inventions" influenced by the Scientific Revolution?
3. What is the contribution of the Scientific Revolution to modern medicine?

● China has its own long and rich history of contributions to science and technology. Among its engineering achievements are the development of matches, the parachute, and the suspension bridge. The Four Great Inventions- the compass, gunpowder, paper-making, and printing- were among the most important technological advancements made. These treasured inventions eventually spread to Western civilization and are still in use today. There were many famous inventors and scientists in the Song Dynasty. The statesman Shen Kou is known for his book *Dream Pool Essay*, in which he wrote about the use of a dry dock to repair boats, the navigational magnetic compass, and the discovery of the concept of true north.

Questions:

1. What is the development of the Four Great Inventions at home and abroad?
2. Could you make a research about Chinese engineering achievements, such as the development of the parachute and the suspension bridge?
3. What is the significance of the book *Dream Pool Essay*?

Part III   Moral Tips

1. Years of effort devoted to understanding the active ingredients of TCM and reformulating classical prescriptions have laid a solid foundation for boosting its role in advancing people's health. TCM treatment also shows promising results in preventing chronic diseases, research conducted in a village in Beijing had shown that combining TCM with Western therapies can play an effective role in preventing colorectal cancer among high-risk populations.

多年来对中药有效成分的研究和对经典方剂的改造，为进一步发挥中医药促进人民健康的作用奠定了坚实基础。中医药治疗在预防慢性疾病方面也显示出良好的效果，在北京一个村庄进行的一项研究表明，在高危人群中，中西医结合可以有效预防大肠癌。

2. Local institutions have assembled first-rate personnel from in and outside China to collaborate on research projects. It was those years of hard work away from the spotlight that have produced the major results of so many research projects today.

地方科研机构汇集了国内外一流人才，共同开展科研项目。正是那些远离聚光灯的艰苦工作，才有了今天这么多研究项目的主要成果。

3. In previous years, we were quite happy about the low-end application of the information and telecom technology, even very proud of the "new four inventions", namely, e-commerce, mobile payment, bicycle-sharing and high-speed rail. Mass innovation and mass entrepreneurship was the slogan which encouraged large numbers of low-end, capital-driven start-ups. Thanks to all the advancements in science and technology made so far, the quality of our lives has improved in many different ways. Science is essential for the well-being and development of all societies.

前几年，我们对信息通信技术的低端应用非常满意，甚至对电子商务、移动支付、共享单车、高铁等"新四大发明"感到非常自豪。"万众创新、大众创业"的口号鼓励了大量低端资本驱动的初创企业。迄今为止科学技术的进步，使得我们的生活质量在许多方面都得到了改善。因此，科学对所有社会的福祉和发展而言都至关重要。

Part IV   Vocabulary Treasure

1. **transform**   *v.*   to competely change the form or appearance or character of sth.

   Using the latest technologies for cooling and heat recovery, we **transform** data centers from energy consumers to sources of sustainable energy.

   利用最新的冷却和热回收技术，我们将数据中心从消耗能源转变为提供可持续能源。

2. **formulate**   *v.*   to create or prepare sth. carefully, giving particular attention to the details

   A statement released after the annual Central Economic Work Conference in December said that China will seize time to **formulate** an action plan for peaking carbon dioxide emissions before 2030.

   12 月中央经济工作会议后发表的一份声明说，中国将抓紧时间制定一项行动计划，争取在 2030 年前实现二氧化碳排放的峰值。

3. **motivated**   *adj.*   inspired; being caused to act in a particular way

   Dai Wen, a doctoral candidate from Tsinghua University's School of Aerospace Engineering, said she felt very excited and **motivated** after watching the livestream.

   来自清华大学航天航空学院的博士生戴文表示，看完直播后，她感到非常兴奋和有动力。

4. **astronomy**   *n.*   the scientific study of the stars, planets, and other natural objects in space

   Besides the technical difficulties, the pair has burned the midnight oil on many nights to study related theories, reading papers on mathematics, physics, chemistry and **astronomy** from home and abroad to gain theoretical support.

除了技术上的困难，两人还在许多个夜晚熬夜学习相关理论，阅读国内外数学、物理、化学、天文学等方面的论文，获得理论支持。

5. **essential**   *adj.*   extremely important or absolutely necessary to a particular subject, situation, or activity

He added that doing a proper warm-up and using the right equipment are both **essential**. Whether one chooses a slope for beginners or for veterans depends on one's skill and physical strength.

他补充说，适当的热身和使用正确的装备都是必要的。选择斜坡是给初学者还是给老手，要看一个人的技巧和体力。

Part V   Language Practice

1. Translate the following paragraph into Chinese.

Reading makes a full man, conference a ready man, and writing an exact man. And therefore, if a man write little, he had need have a great memory; if he confer little, he had need have a present wit; and if he read little, he had need have more cunning, to seem to know that he doth not. Histories make men wise; poets, witty; the mathematics, subtile; natural philosophy, deep; moral, grave; logic and rhetoric, able to contend.

2. Critical thinking

This part is to improve the critical thinking ability by writing a composition.

Directions: Write a composition on the topic: What science has brought to us? The composition is based on the following information, and it is at least 120 words.

➢ **convenience, efficiency and development**

> ➢ **pollution and crisis**
> ➢ **my opinion**

Part VI Further Reading

Nations step up Space cooperation

Scientists from Saudi Arabia will soon have the opportunity to carry out an experiment aboard China's Tiangong space station that is expected to help with the design and production of high-efficiency solar cells.

According to an agreement signed in March 2021 by the Saudi Space Commission and China Manned Space Agency, the Saudi experiment will focus on studying the effects of cosmic rays on the performance of high-efficiency solar cells.

Two institutions from Saudi Arabia, the National Center for Nanotechnology and Advanced Materials and King Abdulaziz City for Science and Technology, are involved in the project, which is among the first nine international science programs selected by the United Nations Office for Outer Space Affairs and China Manned Space Agency to be conducted on board the Tiangong station.

The experiment will aim to improve the efficiency of solar cells operating for long periods to provide a continuous energy supply to satellites and spacecraft, and will also help to reduce the costs of space missions, according to Saudi researchers.

As one of the largest space-based assets mankind has ever deployed in outer space, the Tiangong station currently consists of the Tianhe core module, the Wentian and Mengtian lab modules, the Shenzhou XV spacecraft and the Tianzhou 5 cargo ship.

This massive orbiting outpost has so far received four groups of Chinese astronauts. Currently aboard the station are the three crew members of the Shenzhou XV mission, who arrived on Nov 30 to take over from the Shenzhou

XIV mission.

Tiangong, which has an overall weight of nearly 100 metric tons, is expected to operate in orbit for about 10 years as a space-based platform for science and technology. It will be open to foreign astronauts in the near future, according to Chinese space officials.

China and Saudi Arabia have been engaged in cooperation on space science and technology.

During China's ongoing Chang'e 4 mission, which continues to make the world's first on-site exploration of the far side of the moon, an optical imager developed by Saudi researchers had obtained many pictures of the moon. Moreover, two Saudi satellites have also been launched by China.

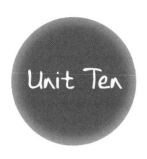

Unit Ten

Virtue of Great Physicians

Bian Que was a legendary Chinese physician who lived during the Warring States period (475—221 BCE). He was known for his extraordinary medical skills and is considered one of the founders of traditional Chinese medicine. According to legend, Bian Que had supernatural abilities and was able to diagnose illnesses just by looking at a patient's face or feeling his pulse.

Bian Que is said to have cured many difficult cases and was particularly famous for his ability to revive the dead. One story tells of how he was able to bring a prince back to life after he had been dead for three days. Bian Que's medical knowledge was also recorded in several ancient texts, including the *Huangdi's Inner Canon*, which is still considered a fundamental text of traditional Chinese medicine.

In addition to his medical achievements, Bian Que was also known for his ethical teachings, which emphasized the importance of treating patients with compassion and respect. His legacy has had a lasting impact on Chinese medicine and his name remains well-known in China today.

Questions:

1. Are you impressed after reading Bian Que's story?

2. Do you know the traditional Chinese medical ways, that is, Four Methods of Diagnosis which was first used and systematized by Bian Que?

3. Do you know any other stories about Bian Que?

Part II   Reading Task

• **Very few scientists can say that four million people are alive because of their work**, but Robert Edwards is one of those few. His development of the technique at the heart of that claim—in vitro fertilization (IVF)—has won him this year's Nobel Prize in Physiology or Medicine.

Questions:

1. Do you know what is "Nobel Prize in Physiology or Medicine"?

2. Can you name any medical scientists in China who won Nobel Prize in Physiology or Medicine?

3. What's the contribution of the winners of Nobel Prize in Physiology or Medicine to the world?

• The expression "basic ethical principles" refers to those general judgements that serve as a basic justification for the many particular ethical prescriptions and evaluations of human actions. Three basic principles, among those generally accepted in our cultural tradition, are particularly relevant to the ethics of research involving human subjects: the principles of respect of persons, beneficence and justice.

Questions:

1. What is the principle of respect for persons?

2. What concrete examples can be given to illustrate the principle of justice?

3. What is the principle of beneficence related to Oath for a Medical Student?

● Patients often complain that their doctors don't listen. Although there are probably a few doctors who truly are tone-deaf, most are reasonably empathic human beings, and I wonder why even these doctors seem prey to this criticism.

Questions:

1. Do you know what's the meaning of the word "empathic" and what's the noun form of the word?

2. To be an empathic doctor, what should he/she do, especially to his/her patients, according to your understanding?

3. To be empathic medical students, what kind of training do you think they can receive in medical schools?

● Soon after I finished my surgical training, I worked with a young doctor who was impressive not only for his clinical skills but also for his devotion to patients. He was large and powerfully built but never seemed to loom over his patients, miraculously shrinking down to their eye level whenever he spoke with them. He listened intently to every detail of their travails and always ended the visits by asking if they still had any unanswered questions.

Questions:

1. What does the phrase "listened intently" mean, especially to a patient?

2. What kind of doctor do you think he was in the above passage?

3. What can we learn from the young doctor dealing with physician-patient relationship?

● First, a physician must be caring. "The secret of the care of the patient is in caring for the patient." There are many texts that describe in eloquent terms the value that patients place on being truly cared for by a physician.

Questions:

1. Why must a physician be caring?
2. How to be caring for a patient?
3. What does the sentence "The secret of the care of the patient is in caring for the patient" mean?

Part III   Moral Tips

1. According to Tu Youyou, the discovery of artemisinin was a team effort. Upon hearing that she had been awarded the Nobel Prize, she said, "The honour is not just mine. There is a team behind me, and all the people of my country. This success proves the great value of traditional Chinese medicine. It is indeed an honour for China's scientific research and Chinese medicine to be spread around the world."

屠呦呦说，青蒿素的发现是一个团队努力的结果。当听到自己被授予诺贝尔奖时，她说："这个荣誉不仅仅属于我。在我身后有一个团队，还有我的国家的全体人民。这一成功证明了中医的巨大价值。中国的科学研究和中医药走向世界，确实是一种荣誉。"

2. The principle of justice means that subjects are selected fairly and that the risks and benefits of research are distributed equitably. Investigators should take precautions not to systematically select subjects simply because of the subjects' easy availability, their compromised position, or because of racial, sexual, economic, or cultural biases in society. Investigators should base inclusion and exclusion criteria on those factors that most effectively and soundly address the

research problem.

公正原则意味着公平地选择研究对象，公平地分配研究的风险和收益。研究人员应采取预防措施，不要仅仅因为受试者容易找到、容易妥协，或者因为社会中的种族、性别、经济或文化偏见而系统地选择受试者。研究者应将纳入其中和排除在外的标准建立在那些最有效和最合理地解决研究问题的因素上。

3. Scholars have postulated several candidates: development of the clinical imagination, deepening of empathy for patients, awareness of the ethical dimensions of clinical situations, and the development of the capacity for attention have all been suggested as the clinical dividends of narrative training.

学者们提出了几种设想：提高临床想象力，加深对患者的共情，认识临床情境叙事维度，培养注意力，这些都被认为是叙事训练所产生的临床益处。

4. To attend gravely and silently, absorbing diastolically what the other says, connotes, displays, performs, and means is required of effective diagnostic and therapeutic work. By emptying the self and by accepting the patient's perspectives and stance, the clinician can allow himself or herself to be filled with the patient's own particular suffering, thereby getting to glimpse the sufferer's needs and desires, as it were, from the inside.

为了达到严肃、静默的关注，有效的诊断和治疗工作要求舒张地吸收他人的话语、暗示、展示、表现和意义。通过清空自我，接受患者的观点和立场，临床医生能够让自己盛满患者的苦难，因此，能够从内心了解患者的需要和欲望。

5. We clinicians donate ourselves as meaning-making vessels to the patient who tells of his or her situation; we act almost as ventriloquists to give voice to that which the patient emits. I put it that way because the patient cannot always tell, in logical or organized language, that which must be told. Instead, these messages come to us through the patient's words, silences, gestures, facial

expressions, and bodily postures as well as physical findings, diagnostic images, and laboratory measurements, and it is our task to cohere these different and sometimes contradictory sources of information so as to create at least provisional meaning.

我们临床医生倾听患者讲述时，要将自己献出，作为意义产生的容器。我们好像是会腹语的人，帮助患者发出声音。之所以这样说，是因为患者并不总是能以有逻辑或有组织的语言讲述自己要说的话，这些信息是通过患者的言语、沉默、手势、面部表情、姿势形体以及体检结果、影像诊断和实验室数据传达到我们这里的。我们的任务是将这些不同的、有时甚至是互相矛盾的信息来源有逻辑地整合在一起，暂时创造出意义。

Part IV Vocabulary Treasure

1. **strive** *v.* try hard to achieve something
   Hold high the great banner of socialism with Chinese characteristics and **strive** in unity to build a modern socialist country in all respects.
   高举中国特色社会主义伟大旗帜，为全面建设社会主义现代化国家而团结奋斗。

2. **patriotic** *adj.* showing love for your country and being proud of it
   We will further advance the Healthy China Initiative and **patriotic** health campaigns and promote sound, healthy lifestyles
   我们将深入开展健康中国行动和爱国卫生运动，倡导文明健康生活方式。

3. **rejuvenation** *n.* the phenomenon of vitality and freshness being restored
   We have developed well-conceived and complete strategic plans for advancing the cause of the Party and the country in the new era. We have put forward the Chinese Dream of the great **rejuvenation** of the

Chinese nation and proposed promoting national rejuvenation through a Chinese path to modernization.

我们对新时代党和国家事业发展作出科学完整的战略部署，提出实现中华民族伟大复兴的中国梦，以中国式现代化推进中华民族伟大复兴。

4. **wellbeing** *n.* a contented state of being happy and healthy and prosperous

In the face of these acute problems and challenges, which undermined the Party's long-term governance, the security and stability of the country, and the **wellbeing** of the people, the Party Central Committee fully assessed the situation, made resolute decisions, and took firm steps.

面对这些影响党长期执政、国家长治久安、人民幸福安康的突出矛盾和问题，党中央审时度势、果敢抉择，锐意进取、攻坚克难。

5. **persistent** *adj.* determined to do sth despite difficulties, especially when other people are against you and think that you are being annoying or unreasonable

We have achieved moderate prosperity, the millennia-old dream of the Chinese nation, through **persistent** hard work. With this, we have elevated China to a higher historical starting point in development.

我们经过接续奋斗，实现了小康这个中华民族的千年梦想，我国发展站在了更高历史起点上。

Part V   Language Practice

1. Translate the following oath into English.

余谨以至诚宣誓：

终身纯洁，忠贞职守。

勿为有损之事，

勿取服或故用有害之药。

尽力提高护理之标准，

慎守病人家务及秘密。

竭诚协助医生之诊治，

勿谋病者之福利。

2. Critical Thinking

This part is to improve the critical thinking ability by writing a composition.

Direction: Write a composition on the topic: **Virtue of Great Physicians.** *The composition is based on the following information, and it is at least 120 words.*

> ➢ **excellent medical skills**
>
> ➢ **noble medical ethics**
>
> ➢ **my opinion**

Part VI   Further Reading

1. Oath for a Medical Student

Health entrusted. Lives confided.

On my admission to the Practice of Medicine, I swear to fulfill, to the best of my ability and judgment, this oath:

I will dedicate myself to medicine with love for my motherland and loyalty to the people.

I will scrupulously practice my profession with conscience and dignity.

I will discipline myself and give my teachers the respect and gratitude that is their due.

I will strive diligently for continued excellence and my full development.

I will do my utmost to alleviate human suffering and promote human health, safeguarding the sanctity and honor of medicine.

I will heal the wounded and rescue the dying regardless of the trials and tribulations.

As long as my life endures, may I commit myself to advance the nation's medical science and research as well as the well-being of the entire human race.

2. Compendium of Materia Medica by Li Shizhen

Li Shizhen (1518—1593) was a distinguished doctor of the Ming Dynasty. He spent 27 years writing the most complete guide to medicines of ancient China entitled *Compendium of Materia Medica*.

In 1556, Li Shizhen was appointed the chief director of the Imperial Medical Institute, which had medical books from all dynasties and provided Li Shizhen with new insights. One day, doctors in the Imperial Medical Institute were discussing official business. Li Shizhen suggested, "Commissioner, the *Materia Medica* hasn't been revised for several hundred years. The old *Materia Medica* has too many mistakes. Please send a memorial to the emperor, suggesting the old *Materia Medica* be revised." The commissioner said: "The Imperial Medical Institute is to serve the emperor. At present, it is short of money to refine the pills of immortality. How can we spend so much effort and money in revising the *Materia Medica*?" Li Shizhen was so angry that he resigned from his post by the excuse of sickness and returned to his hometown. Unexpectedly, Li Shizhen's father, who was also a doctor, died several months ago. His father left Li Shizhen with a dozen medical books that might be needed in revising the *Materia Medica*. Li Shizhen made up his mind to rivise the *Materia Medica* although the imperial court refused to support him.

People from all sides contributed their prescriptions, which greatly inspired Li Shizhen. At night, Li Shizhen checked, reedited and categorized the prescriptions and herbal medicines in accordance with the medical books. Since 1565, Li Shizhen, with innumerable questions about the ancient *Materia Medica*, started his ten-year expedition. Li Shizhen and his followers walked thousands of miles, mastering a lot of information which was needed for the revision of the book. Finally they arrived home. Li Shizhen divided the medical information gathered into 16 parts and 60 categories according to plant, animal, mineral and the like, which broke down the method of classification in the past according to the grade of herbal medicines: superior, middle and inferior. This approach was very close to the contemporary scientific classification principle. Li Shizhen wrote down the name, producing area, shape, cultivating and collecting method, smell and function of each medicine component in detail and enclosed the shape sketch of each medicine.

After 27 years of hard work, at the age of 61, Li Shizhen finally completed the monumental work entitled the *Compendium of Materia Medica*. In 1596, the *Compendium of Materia Medica* came out, causing a great stir. Bookstores all over the country made copies of the book one after another. It became a great classic work of Chinese medicine. By then, Li Shizhen had been dead for three years. Later, the book, reputed as the great medical work in the Orient, was translated into many languages.

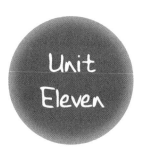

Ecological Civilization

Part I Pre-Reading Task

On August 24, 2021, Chinese President Xi Jinping inspected Saihanba Forest Farm in north China's Hebei Province. Saihanba is considered to be a miracle as it has been transformed from barren land to lush forest through the extraordinary efforts of three generations of Chinese people.

Saihanba was previously been home to abundant forest resources and high biodiversity 400 years ago. With a cool summer and lush vegetation, the area was set to be a royal retreat. However, deforestation and constant wars turned the area into a desert by the end of the Qing Dynasty (1644—1911). As the forest barrier was gone, sandstorms became more frequent. To stop sandstorms that kept threatening or event striking Beijing, Tianjin and other northern China cities, the Forestry Administration decided in 1962 to set the Saihanba Mechanical Forest Farm, and sent 369 foresters, mostly in their 20s, to the area for tree planting.

The first group of foresters in Saihanba faced many challenges, equipped with only the simplest tools amid extreme coldness and drought. As result, they were unable to ensure the survival of trees planted. However, after the joint efforts of three generations, Saihanba was restored and turned back into a green paradise with a forest coverage raised from 11.4 percent to 80 percent, which can conserve and purify 137 million cubic meters of water every year.

The miraculous planting story of foresters in Saihanba gives rise to the concept of the Saihanba Spirit, defined as working hard, advancing against difficulties, forging ahead, and innovating boldly. As one of the largest man-made plantations in the world, the Saihanba Afforestation Community won the honor of Champions of the Earth in 2017 due to the efforts to transform degraded land into a green paradise. Now, the lush Saihanba has become home to thousands of species of flora and fauna for its good environment, and also attracts numerous tourists.

Questions:

1. Give a brief summary of the story and spirit of Saihanba.
2. Share with your classmates what you have learned from this article.
3. What other efforts do you know China has made in preserving natural resources during the past decades?

Part II   Reading Task

- "It's a satisfying life too. In the summer we canoe on the river, go picnicking in the woods and take long bicycle rides. In the winter we ski and skate. We get excited about sunsets. We love the smell of earth warming and the sound of cattle lowing. We watch for hawks in the sky and deer in the cornfields."

Questions:

1. What do you think of the life and scene described in this paragraph?
2. What is your dream lifestyle?
3. Do you think man should live in harmony with nature?

- "... The trade in endangered animals is on the increase. For example, a thousand rhinos will be shot in South Africa this year because their horns are used in alternative medicine. UK customs officials have confiscated 2.5 million items, 10 times more than the year before. They include 4,000 kilos of illegally imported medicines, 93 endangered live animals, such as reptiles, tortoises and turtles, and over 300 items made from ivory. the items are sent by post or by courier and are intercepted at UK ports and airports. Endangered animals brought in alive are re-homed across the country, but tortoises and turtles in particular are difficult to find homes for. Education and research benefit from many of the items, but the rhino horn will be destroyed, to stop it going back onto the black market."

Questions:

1. Do you agree that the trade in endangered animals should be illegal? Why or why not?
2. What measures has China taken to protect endangered animals?
3. Should museums and universities be allowed to keep some items for education and research purposes? Why or why not?

● "The importance of biodiversity seems obvious to us. We enjoy the beauty of biodiversity when we take a walk in the park, take a trip to the zoo or a wild area, read books or watch TV shows about strange creatures in foreign lands. Some people believe that biodiversity is important simply because it is so wonderful. Some think there are philosophical or spiritual reasons for biodiversity. But there are other reasons why it is so important.

The loss of biodiversity will change the balance of life on Earth. If an ecosystem is destroyed, many species adapted to that ecosystem may very likely be destroyed as well. If that species is what scientists call "keystone", a whole ecosystem may depend on it. Biodiversity is also important in its direct benefits to people. Plants give us the air we breathe; animals and plants supply us with the food we eat; and organisms and microorganisms clean the air, regulate floods, recycle waste, and control pests.

Biodiversity also has economic and health benefits. Both industry and agriculture depend on it for raw material and other things. And medicine is even more dependent on biodiversity. In China, more than 5,000 species of plants are used for medicinal purposes. May species which were thought "useless" at first are found to be valuable. And this is a further threat from the loss of biodiversity."

Questions:

1. Do you know anything about biological diversity or biodiversity?
2. What has China been doing to control environmental pollution?
3. What are the effective outcomes of Chinese pollution control?

Part III Moral Tips

1. For I am abstracted from the world, the world from nature, nature from the way, and the way from what is beneath abstraction.

人法地，地法天，天法道，道法自然。

——老子

2. Heaven, Earth, and I were produced together, and all things and I are one.

天地与我并生，而万物与我为一，天人合一。

——庄子

3. Major projects for preserving and restoring key ecosystems will be carried out at a faster pace in priority areas, including key national ecosystem service zones, ecological conservation redlines, and nature reserves.

以国家重点生态功能区、生态保护红线、自然保护地等为重点，加快实施重要生态系统保护和修复重大工程。

4. Enhancing diversity, stability, and sustainability in our eco-systems.

提升生态系统多样性、稳定性、持续性。

Part IV Vocabulary Treasure

1. **prosperous** *adj.* in fortunate circumstances financially; rich and successful

   Over the past five years, we have continued to strengthen the overall leadership of the Party and the centralized, unified leadership of the Central Committee. We have devoted great energy to finishing building a moderately **prosperous** society in all respects.

   五年来，我们坚持加强党的全面领导和党中央集中统一领导，全力推进全面建成小康社会进程。

2. **harmony** *n.* a state of peaceful existence and agreement

   We stepped up law-based administration, promoted social advancement, and safeguarded social **harmony** and stability.

   加强依法行政和社会建设，保持社会和谐稳定。

3. **sustainable** *adj.* that can continue or be continued for a long time

   A review of our respective progress in economic and social development shows that China and Saudi Arabia have so much in common: Both countries have followed development paths suited to their national conditions; both of us have achieved future-oriented **sustainable** economic development in diverse ways; and both countries have endeavored to improve our people's lives.

   纵观中沙各自的经济社会发展进程，我们发现，两国都立足国情，走适合自身的发展道路；都着眼长远，推进经济可持续和多元化发展；都以人为本，不断提高人民生活水平。

4. **ecological** *adj.* characterized by the interdependence of living organisms in an environment; of or relating to the science of ecology

   The Communist Party of China Central Committee and the State Council have jointly issued an outline document on the **ecological** protection and high-quality development of the Yellow River basin.

中共中央和国务院近日印发《黄河流域生态保护和高质量发展规划纲要》。

5. **integrity**   *n.*   the quality of being honest and having strong moral principles; (formal) the state of being whole and not divided

Wc will strengthen the professional **integrity**, conduct, and ability of our teachers, foster public respect for educators, and encourage public support for education.

加强师德师风建设，培养高素质教师队伍，弘扬尊师重教社会风尚。

All countries should respect each other's sovereignty, dignity and territorial **integrity**, each other's development paths and social systems, and each other's core interests and major concerns.

各国应尊重彼此主权、尊严、领土完整，尊重彼此发展道路和社会制度，尊重彼此核心利益和重大关切。

Part V   Language Practice

1. Translate the following paragraph into English.

传统农业以精耕细作著称于世。在长期实践中人们认识到农业生产的运作必须与气候季节变化的节奏保持一致，"不违农时"成为人们的共识，并逐步形成以二十四节气为中心的综合运用物候、天象、气象等多种手段的农业指时体系。土地是农业生产的物质载体，先民们很早就认识到"因地制宜"的重要性，强调综合运用耕作、施肥和灌溉等措施，为作物生长创造良好的土壤环境。夏商周时期，出现了畎亩结合的土地利用方式；春秋战国至魏晋南北朝，创造了灵活多样的轮作倒茬和间作套种方式；隋唐宋元，水稻与麦类等水旱轮作一年两熟的复种有了初步的发展；明清，又出现了建立在综合利用（多层次循环利用）水土、生物资源基础上的立体农业（生态农业）的雏形。用地与养地结合，使"地力常新"。这些举措都渗透了我国古代"天人合一"的哲学思想。

2. Critical Thinking

This part is to improve the critical thinking ability by writing a composition.

Direction: Over the past few years, we have witnessed disasters caused by human activities. As a university student, please write a composition on the topic: A Letter of Appeal to raise people's awareness of these natural disasters and the protection of the environment. The composition is based on the following information, and it is at least 120 words.

> ➢ **give examples of natural disasters caused by human activities**
> ➢ **propose some necessary precautions**
> ➢ **call everyone to take action to save the Earth**

Part VI   Further Reading

1. Yangtze River: The mother river needs to heal (excerpt)

The Yangtze River, China's mother river, has been going through a transformation since the general principle of replacing exploitation with protection was laid out in 2012. A policy of no large-scale development projects has been put in place, while restoring the ecology and improving the environment has been made a top national priority. Measures including pollution control and a 10-year fishing ban have been established across 11 provinces and municipalities along the Yangtze River.

Behind the efforts is the urgency to protect the Yangtze, which has been ailing because of pollution, overfishing, sand dredging and other exploitative activities.

...

Better Yangtze, better economy

The Yangtze is China's longest waterway and the world's busiest inner waterway in terms of cargo flow. The Yangtze River Economic Belt, which generates about half of the country's GDP, is home to many of the country's free trade zones, playing an important role in coordinating the opening up of coastal, river, border and inland areas.

Take the Yangtze River Delta as an example. The delta, located on the eastern and coastal end of the economic belt, encompasses Shanghai and the provinces of Jiangsu, Zhejiang and Anhui in East China. Roughly the size of Germany, it is one of China's most economically active, open and innovative regions thanks to fast-paced regional integration. It brings together all kinds of enterprises that play important parts in the global industry chains of automobiles, semiconductors and photovoltaics.

Chinese President Xi Jinping urged for high-quality development of the Yangtze River Economic Belt at a symposium in November 2020, stressing the importance of green development, which integrates regional economic development with ecological conservation.

The approach is designed to build the Belt into a powerful engine of the country's development, bringing more certainty to the development of the world economy.

Despite these efforts, the Yangtze's protection remains a difficult task. When a new action plan to further combat pollution and restore biodiversity of the Yangtze by the end of 2025 was announced in September, the Ministry of Ecology and Environment said that breakthroughs are needed in the preservation and rehabilitation of the aquatic ecology, and the general situation of the Yangtze remains complex, leaving a daunting challenge.

2. China's ecological vision a key input to global governance (excerpt)

Global environmental governance reached a crossroads as climate change, biodiversity losses and ocean pollution pose direct threats to the ecosystem and human well-being, affecting food, health and security, the global priority continues to be shifted to ramping up fossil fuel production, amid sharply rising geo-political tensions, to secure supply for post-pandemic economic recoveries.

Breaking this impasse needs both visionary thinking and creative solutions.

As the second largest economy in the world, China's pursuit of ecological civilization has naturally caught the attention of the world.

Ecological civilization contains a broad and profound theory. It means building a new form of civilization that enables man and nature to coexist harmoniously. Recognizing that the earth is so far the only planet in the known universe that has life and that nature itself is fundamental for the entire humanity to live and to prosper, eco-civilization calls for respecting, adapting to and protecting nature in any social-economic development.

Eco-civilization has its roots in rich ancient Chinese philosophy and culture, such as Confucianism, Taoism, and Buddhism, which advocate balance, moderation and respect for nature. It also draws inspiration from modern environmental theories and practices, such as sustainability, inclusive development, circular economy and low-carbon transition.

Eco-civilization is not only a concept. To put it into practice, eco-civilization was written into China's constitution in 2018. Following its guidance, China launched massive clean air and clean water action plans, by building tens of thousands of monitoring stations across the country and vastly strengthening environmental enforcement. Besides, China achieved a great improvement in air quality in the world, with Beijing's PM2.5 concentration dropping by 66.5 percent from 2013 to 2022.

Also last year, China's GDP topped 120 trillion Chinese yuan($17.24 trillion). China's economic development has achieved tremendous success and provided by far a major contribution to global economic growth, which boosts confidence for China to pursue concerted efforts to cut carbon emissions, reduce pollution, expand green development and pursue higher-quality economic growth.

China's ecological concept and practices could help create innovative solutions to address global challenges. At the international level, China has actively participated in global environmental governance and cooperation. To tackle climate change, China has ratified the Paris Agreement, building the world's largest solar and wind power capacity, and cut its carbon intensity by more than one-third and the share of coal in primary energy consumption dropped from 68.5 percent to 56 percent in the past 10 years. China has committed to peak its carbon dioxide emissions by 2030 and achieve carbon neutrality by 2060.

To address biodiversity losses, China hosted the United Nations Biodiversity Conference (COP15) in 2022 and made a great contribution to ensure its success. Biodiversity draws increasingly greater attention from the international community as it is under serious threat globally. With the world population more than doubling and global GDP growing from $3.4 trillion in 1970 to $85.3 trillion by 2020, nature has suffered enormous losses in half a century as the global population of mammals, birds, amphibians, reptiles and fish declining by two-thirds on average, concluded by the Living Planet Report 2020.

From 2022, China has embarked on a new journey to pursue a Chinese path to modernization, with harmonious coexistence between man and nature an integral part of it. It will help further develop eco-civilization in China's long-term social-economic development. It will also enable China to make more input in global environmental governance and to provide more support to other countries, particularly the global south, in their pursuits of sustainable development and common prosperity for all.

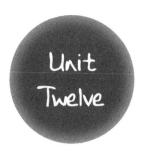

Unit
Twelve

Natural Harmony

The Great Smog of London, lethal smog that covered the city of London for five days (December 5—9) in 1952, caused by a combination of industrial pollution and high-pressure weather conditions. This combination of smoke and fog brought the city to a near standstill and resulted in thousands of deaths. Its consequences prompted the passing of the Clean Air Act four years later, which marked a turning point in the history of environmentalism.

The Great Smog of 1952 was a pea-souper of unprecedented severity, induced by both weather and pollution. On the whole, during the 20th century, the fogs of London had become more infrequent, as factories began to migrate outside the city. However, on December 5, an anticyclone settled over London, a high-pressure weather system that caused an inversion whereby cold air was trapped below warm air higher up. Consequently, the emissions of factories and domestic fires could not be released into the atmosphere and remained trapped near ground level. The result was the worst pollution-based fog in the city's history.

Visibility was so impaired in some parts of London that pedestrians were unable to see their own feet. Aside from the Underground, transportation was severely restricted. Ambulance services suffered, leaving people to find their own way to hospitals in the smog. Many people simply abandoned their cars on the road. Indoor plays and concerts were cancelled as audiences were unable to see the stage, and crime on the streets increased. There was a spike in deaths and hospitalizations relating to pneumonia and bronchitis, and herds of cattle in Smithfield reportedly choked to death. Though the fog lasted five days, the effects of the smog were long-lasting, however, and present-day estimates rank the number of deaths to have been about 12,000.

Questions:

1. What was the Great Smog of London in 1952 caused by?
2. What were the effects of the Great Smog of London?
3. Why is its consequence said to be a turning point in the history of environmentalism?

Part II   Reading Task

• There was once a town where all life seemed to live in harmony with its surroundings. The town lay in the midst of a checkerboard of prosperous farms, with fields of grain and hillsides of orchards where, in spring, white clouds of bloom drifted above the green fields. In autumn, oak and maple and birch set up a blaze of colour that flamed and flickered across a backdrop of pines. Then foxes barked in the hills and deer silently crossed the fields, half hidden in the mists of the autumn mornings.

Along the road, laurel viburnum and alder, great ferns and wild flowers, delighted the travellers' eyes through much of the year. Even in winter the roadsides were places of beauty, where countless birds came to feed on the berries and on the seed heads of the dried weeds rising above the snow. The countryside was, in fact, famous for the abundance and variety of its bird life, and when the flood of migrants was pouring through in spring and autumn people travelled from great distances to observe them. Others came to fish the streams, which flowed clear and cold out of the hills and contained shady pools where trout lay.

> **Questions:**
> 1. What kind of life do people live in the town?
> 2. What do you think of the environment or ecosystem described in the paragraphs?
> 3. Do you think ecosystems are essential for the world?

- In the gutters under the eaves and between the shingles of the roofs, white granular power still showed a few patches; some weeks before it had fallen like snow upon the roofs and the lawns, the fields and streams.

No witchcraft, no enemy action had silenced the rebirth of new life in this stricken world. The people had done it themselves.

> **Questions:**
> 1. Please paraphrase the sentence "No witchcraft, no enemy action had silenced the rebirth of new life in this stricken world. The people had done it themselves."
> 2. According to the writer, what would happen to new life if the world were stricken by disasters?
> 3. What did the writer think had caused the disasters in the world?

- Hero to the Homeless

For more than 20 years, Dr. Jim Withers has been providing medical care to homeless people in Pittsburgh. To gain their trust and develop a connection with them, Withers was dressed like a homeless person, with dirty clothes and dirty hair. Then he searched on the streets, in the alleys and under bridges for people who needed medical care.

Questions:

1. What has Dr. Jim Withers been doing during the 20 years?
2. Why did Dr. Jim Withers dress himself like a homeless person?
3. Do you think we need to help the poor and needy people and to give them a hand up?

● Water is on track to be the most important and most contentious resource of the 21st century. It could replace oil as the strategic resource that triggers geopolitical conflicts. But with the right solutions, it could also be the one that brings us all together.

Questions:

1. What has caused heated arguments about water?
2. According to the writer, what conflicts might arise?
3. What does the writer think might be a right solution to unite people around the world?

● The reason energy and water sit at the top, ahead of food and poverty, is that addressing them makes subsequent problems easier to deal with. Developing abundant sources of clean, reliable, affordable energy enables an abundance of clean water. An abundance of clean water enables food production and protects the environment.

Questions:

1. Why do energy and water rank the top of the crises, above food and poverty?
2. What is the relationship between energy and water?
3. Will abundant source of energy and water help to protect the environment?

Part III   Moral Tips

1. This beautiful land of China, home to the Chinese nation and its splendid 5,000-year civilization, has nurtured the lofty idea of harmony between man and nature.

锦绣中华大地，是中华民族赖以生存和发展的家园，孕育了中华民族 5 000 多年的灿烂文明，造就了中华民族天人合一的崇高追求。

2. Ecological conservation has become part of China's overall plan for national development. Building a beautiful China is an inspiring goal for the Chinese people. As China steps up its conservation efforts, the world will see a China with more blue skies, lush mountains and lucid waters.

现在，生态文明建设已经纳入中国国家发展总体布局，建设美丽中国已经成为中国人民心向往之的奋斗目标。中国生态文明建设进入了快车道，天更蓝、山更绿、水更清将不断展现在世人面前。

3. The history of civilizations shows that the rise or fall of a civilization is closely tied to its relationship with nature. Industrialization, while generating unprecedented material wealth, has incurred serious damage to Mother Nature. Development without thought to the future is not sustainable. The way forward should be green development that focuses on harmony with nature and eco-friendly progress.

纵观人类文明发展史，生态兴则文明兴，生态衰则文明衰。工业化进程创造了前所未有的物质财富，也产生了难以弥补的生态创伤。杀鸡取卵、竭泽而渔的发展方式走到了尽头，顺应自然、保护生态的绿色发展昭示着未来。

4. Looking up at night, we are awed by many stars in the sky. Yet, the planet Earth is the only home for mankind. We must protect this planet like our own eyes, and cherish nature the way we cherish life. We must preserve what gives our planet life and embrace green development.

仰望夜空，繁星闪烁。地球是全人类赖以生存的唯一家园。我们要像保护自己的眼睛一样保护生态环境，像对待生命一样对待生态环境，同筑生态文明之基，同走绿色发展之路！

5. We need to advocate harmony between man and nature. Lush mountains, green fields, singing birds and blossoming flowers offer more than beauty to the eye. They are the basis for future development. Nature will punish those who exploit and plunder it brutally, and reward those who use and protect it carefully. We must maintain the overall balance of the Earth's eco-system, so that our children and children's children will not only have material wealth but also enjoy starry skies, green mountains and sweet flowers.

我们应该追求人与自然的和谐。山峦层林尽染，平原蓝绿交融，城乡鸟语花香。这样的自然美景，既带给人们美的享受，也是人类走向未来的依托。无序开发、粗暴掠夺，人类定会遭到大自然的无情报复；合理利用、友好保护，人类必将获得大自然的慷慨回报。我们要维持地球生态整体平衡，让子孙后代既能享有丰富的物质财富，又能遥望星空、看见青山、闻到花香。

6. I thought I knew a good deal about China, but until I spent weeks among China's poor people and poor counties, I had no idea how targeted poverty alleviation worked. I witnessed five methods of poverty alleviation in action: Creating a small industry (usually agriculture); creating a sustainable micro-business; relocating, moving whole villages from remote areas; education and training; ecological compensation for those living in ecologically vulnerable areas; and social security, medical subsidies and direct payments to those who cannot work.

我以为我对中国很了解，但直到我在中国的贫困县与贫困人口一起待了几个星期，我才知道精准扶贫的效果如何。我亲眼看见了其实施的五种扶贫方法：产业扶贫（通常是农业领域），创立可持续发展的小微企业；对偏远地区的贫困村进行整村搬迁、安置；加强教育和培训；为生活在生态脆弱地区的人们提供生态补偿；加强社会保障、医疗补贴，对无劳动能力的人直接给予补助。

7. Yangtze River Protection Law, passed at the 24th Standing Committee session of the 13th National People's Congress, took effect on March 1, 2021. The law is formulated to strengthen the protection and restoration of the ecological environment in the Yangtze River basin, facilitate the effective and rational use of resources, safeguard ecological security, ensure harmony between human and nature, and achieve the sustainable development of the Chinese nation.

第十三届全国人大常委会第二十四次会议通过的《长江保护法》从 2021 年 3 月 1 日起实施。制定该法是为了加强长江流域生态环境保护和修复，促进资源合理高效利用，保障生态安全，实现人与自然和谐共生、中华民族永续发展。

8. In the face of climate change, which is a major challenge to all humanity, we need to advocate green and low-carbon development, actively promote solar, wind and other sources of renewable energy, work for effective implementation of the Paris Agreement on climate change and keep strengthening our capacity for sustainable development.

面对气候变化这一全人类重大挑战，我们要倡导绿色低碳理念，积极发展太阳能、风能等可再生能源，推动应对气候变化《巴黎协定》有效实施，不断增强可持续发展能力。

Part IV   Vocabulary Treasure

1. **conservation**   *n.*   the protection of plants and animals, natural areas, and interesting and important structures and buildings, especially from the damaging effects of human activity
We will advance the Beautiful China Initiative and take a holistic

and systematic approach to the **conservation** and improvement of mountains, waters, forests, farmlands, grasslands, and deserts.

我们要推进美丽中国建设，坚持山水林田湖草沙一体化保护和系统治理。

2. **civilization**   *n.*   a state of human society that is very developed and organized

Civilizations only vary from each other, just as human beings are different only in terms of skin color and the language used. No civilization is superior over others.

人类只有肤色语言之别，文明只有姹紫嫣红之别，但绝无高低优劣之分。

3. **emission**   *n.*   the act of sending gas, heat, light, etc. out into the air

We will promote concerted efforts to cut carbon **emissions**, reduce pollution, expand green development, and purse economic growth.

我们要协同推进降碳、减污、扩绿、增长。

4. **abundant**   *adj.*   (formal) existing in large quantities; more than enough

A just cause enjoys **abundant** support while an unjust cause finds little support.

得道多助，失道寡助。

5. **preserve**   *v.*   to keep a particular quality, feature, etc.

It is critical to **preserve** one's true nature of benevolence so as to cultivate a genuine self of moral excellence.

保持人之本心，养护人之本性。

6. **exploitation**   *n.*   the use of land, oil, minerals, etc.

We should put more efforts in scientific and technological innovation to raise the technological level of **exploitation** of rare earths, which is strategically important but nonrenewable.

稀土是重要的战略资源，也是不可再生资源。要加大科技创新力度，不断提高开发利用的技术水平。

Part V   Language Practice

1. Translate the following paragraph into English.

目前，全球的环境问题已经严重影响到人类的生存环境。中国作为一个发展中国家，面临着发展经济和保护环境的双重任务。中国从本国国情出发，在全面推进现代化的过程中，将环境保护视为一项基本国策，把实现可持续发展作为一个重大战略，在全国范围内开展了大规模的污染防治和生态环境保护。实践表明，中国实行的经济、社会和环境协调发展的方针是有成效的。

2. Critical Thinking

This part is to improve the critical thinking ability by writing a composition.

Direction: Write a composition on the topic: Effects and Solutions of Water Pollution. The composition is based on the following information, and it is at least 120 words.

> ➢ the common causes of water pollution in your city
> ➢ the reason(s) why water is critical in sustainable development
> ➢ my opinion on solutions taken to balance economic growth and environment protection

Part VI   Further Reading

1. Applying systems thinking and a coordinated approach (excerpt)

Green development is an all-round revolutionary change in our values, and in how we work, live, and think. China has applied systems thinking to the whole process of economic and social development and eco-environmental conservation and protection. It has taken a sound approach to the relationships between development and protection, between overall and local interests, and between the present and the future. It has taken a scientific, moderate, and orderly approach to the use of territorial space, and promoted a sound economic structure that facilitates green, low-carbon, and circular development. It has fostered an institutional system that combines both constraints and incentives to coordinate industrial restructuring, pollution control, eco-environmental conservation, and climate response. China has endeavored to cut carbon emissions, reduce pollution, expand green development, and pursue economic growth. It has prioritized eco-environmental protection, conserves resources and uses them efficiently for green and low-carbon development. It has developed spatial configurations, industrial structures, and ways of work and life that help conserve resources and protect the environment, and promoted greener economic and social development in all respects.

2. Air quality and health

What is air pollution and how does it lead to disease in our bodies?

Air pollution is the presence of one or more contaminants in the atmosphere, such as dust, fumes, gas, mist, odor, smoke or vapor, in quantities and duration that can be injurious to human health. The main pathway of exposure from air pollution is through the respiratory tract. Breathing in these pollutants leads to inflammation, oxidative stress, immunosuppression, and mutagenicity in cells throughout our body, impacting the lungs, heart, brain among other organs and ultimately leading to disease.

What organs are impacted by air pollution?

Almost every organ in the body can be impacted by air pollution. Due to their small size, some air pollutants are able to penetrate into the bloodstream via the lungs and circulate throughout the entire body leading to systemic inflammation and carcinogenicity.

What diseases are associated with exposure to air pollution?

Air pollution is a risk for all-cause mortality as well as specific diseases. The specific disease outcomes most strongly linked with exposure to air pollution include stroke, is chasmic heart disease, chronic obstructive pulmonary disease, lung cancer, pneumonia, and cataract (household air pollution only).

There is suggestive evidence also linking air pollution exposure with increased risk for adverse pregnancy outcomes (i.e. low-birth weight, small for gestational age), other cancers, diabetes, cognitive impairment and neurological diseases.

What are some of the most important air pollutants leading to disease?

Although there are many toxins that have adverse impacts on health, pollutants with the strongest evidence for public health concern include particulate matter (PM), carbon monoxide (CO), ozone (O_3), nitrogen dioxide (NO_2) and Sulphur dioxide (SO_2). Fine particulate matter is an especially important source of health risks, as these very small particles can penetrate deep into the lungs, enter the bloodstream, and travel to organs causing systemic damages to tissues and cells.

How long does someone need to be exposed to air pollution to harm their health?

Health problems in children and adults can occur because of both short- and long-term exposure to air pollutants. The levels and duration of exposure that can be considered 'safe' vary by pollutant, as well as the related disease outcomes. For some pollutants, there are no thresholds below which adverse effects do not occur.

Exposure to high levels of particulate matter, for example, can lead to reduced lung function, respiratory infections and aggravated asthma from short-term exposure. Whereas long-term or chronic exposure to fine particulate matter increases a person's risk for diseases with a longer onset, like some noncommunicable diseases including stroke, heart disease, chronic obstructive pulmonary disease and cancer.

Are some populations more likely to be at higher risk for disease from air pollution?

The children, elderly and pregnant women are more susceptible to air pollution-related diseases. Genetics, comorbidities, nutrition and sociodemographic factors also impact a person's susceptibility to air pollution.

Does exposure to air pollution during pregnancy impact the health of the fetus?

Maternal exposure to air pollution is associated with adverse birth outcomes, such as low birth weight, pre-term birth and small for gestational age births.

A growing body of evidence also suggests that air pollution may affect diabetes and neurological development in children.

Are the health risks the same between ambient air pollution and household air pollution?

The health impacts from exposure to ambient air pollution or household air pollution are dependent on the types and concentrations of the pollutants in the air pollution mixture to which an individual is exposed. However, the health risks and disease pathways between ambient and household air pollution exposure are often similar, due to their similar composition. Fine particulate matter for example is a common and critical pollutant of both ambient and household air pollution leading to negative health impacts.

Additional safety risks are associated with many of the fuels and technologies used in the home emitting air pollution. These include burns and poisonings (from kerosene ingestion), as well as physical injury related to fuel collection, including musculoskeletal damage, violence, and animal bites.

It is important to note that the death and disability estimates attributed to air pollution do not account for all health outcomes associated with air pollution. WHO estimates are likely conservative as only health outcomes for which there is strong certainty in the epidemiological evidence are included (i.e. stroke, ischemic heart disease, chronic obstructive pulmonary disease, pneumonia, and lung cancer).

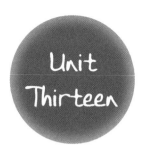

Unit Thirteen

Innovative Awareness

Part I Pre-Reading Task

When it comes to science and technology, there is no limit for the country's scientists to pursue excellence. During his recent inspection trip in Guizhou province, President Xi Jinping met with the project leaders and core scientists of China's Five-hundred-meter Aperture Spherical Radio Telescope (FAST).

FAST, with its unparalleled collecting area, state of art receiver systems, and the digital back-end of which the technology development largely follows the Moore's law, owns a unique window for contribution through precise measurements of matter as well as energy in the low frequency radio band.

Xi, general secretary of the Communist Party of China Central Committee and chairman of the Central Military Commission, recalled scientists to make efforts to scale the heights of global science, secure new achievements in key fields and make greater contributions to developing China's scientific and technological strength at a faster pace and realizing the country's self-reliance and self-improvement in science and technology.

> **Questions:**
> 1. What is of great significance of China's Five-hundred-meter Aperture Spherical Radio Telescope (FAST)?

2. Why should our nation focus more on technological innovation?

3. **Fast** is another name of "**Tian Yan**" in Chinese, and the deification of the eyes in ancient China is inseparable from the ancestor worship of the ancients. Besides, it's the ancients' desire to know the universe and the extension of their inner expectations. Can you list any examples about the link between "**Tian Yan**" and our mythical images?

Part II   Reading Task

● Anyway, even if one wanted to, one couldn't put the clock back to an earlier age. Knowledge and techniques can't just be forgotten. Nor can one prevent further advances in the future.

Questions:

1. What is the definition of an earlier age?

2. How do you like the fact that "knowledge and techniques" bring about advances in technology?

3. What knowledge and techniques can't be forgotten? List the examples.

● Even if all government money for research were cut off (and the present government is doing its best), the force of competition would still bring about advances in technology.

Questions:

1. Why is government money allocated for research?

2. What is the link between the force of competition and advances in technology?

3. How can we promote our awareness of advances in technology?

● Moreover, one cannot stop inquiring minds from thinking about basic science, whether or not they are paid for it. The only way to prevent further developments would be a global state that suppressed anything new, and human initiative and inventiveness are such that even this wouldn't succeed. All it would do is slow down the rate of change.

Questions:
1. How do you like inquiring minds from thinking about basic science?
2. What is the similarity and difference between "inventiveness" and "innovation"?
3. What will slow down the rate of change? List the examples.

● What can be done to harness this interest and give the public the scientific background it needs to make informed decisions on subjects like acid rain, the greenhouse effect, nuclear weapons, and genetic engineering? Clearly, the basis must lie in what is taught in schools.

Questions:
1. Why should the scientific background be given to the public?
2. What does the author list the examples like acid rain, the greenhouse effect, nuclear weapons, and genetic engineering?
3. What should be taught in schools according to the author?

● But in schools, science is often presented in a dry and uninteresting manner. Children learn it by rote to pass examinations, and they don't see its relevance to the world around them. Moreover, science is often taught in terms of equations. Although equations are a brief and accurate way of describing mathematical ideas, they frighten most people.

Questions:

1. What is the importance of acquiring the relevance to the world around the children?

2. Why is science often taught in terms of equations in the schools? List the examples.

3. Since equations are a brief and accurate way of describing mathematical ideas, why do they frighten most people?

● Only television can reach a truly mass audience. There are some very good science programs on TV, but others present scientific wonders simply as magic, without explaining them or showing how they **fit into the framework of scientific ideas**. Producers of television science programs should realize that they have a responsibility to educate the public, not just entertain it.

Questions:

1. What does the author mention that only television can reach a truly mass audience?

2. Why do others present scientific wonders simply as magic?

3. What is the real role of television science programs?

Part III　Moral Tips

1. As strategic partners, China and Arab states should carry forward the spirit of China-Arab friendship, strengthen solidarity and cooperation, and foster a closer China-Arab community with a shared future, so as to deliver greater benefits to our peoples and advance the cause of human progress.

中阿作为战略伙伴，应该继承和发扬中阿友好精神，加强团结合作，构建更加紧密的中阿命运共同体，更好造福双方人民，推动人类进步事业不断向前发展。

2. China should improve the comprehensive management system for intellectual property. China needs to coordinate IPR protection, anti-monopoly, and fair competition reviews to promote the orderly flow and efficient allocation of innovation resources.

中国应该健全知识产权综合管理体制。统筹实施知识产权保护、反垄断、公平竞争审查等工作，促进创新要素自主有序流动、高效配置。

3. In 2013, I put forth the initiative to jointly build a Silk Road Economic Belt and a 21st Century Maritime Silk Road. Six years on, with the concerted efforts of many partics, we have developed a plan for advancing Belt and Road cooperation and reaped many benefits.

2013 年，我提出共建丝绸之路经济带和 21 世纪海上丝绸之路的倡议。六年来，在各方的共同努力下，我们制定了推进"一带一路"合作的计划，取得了丰硕成果。

4. Promote innovation-driven development and the digital economy. Innovation is an important driving force that propels world development. We need to commit ourselves to innovation-driven development, harness the power of the digital economy as a new growth engine, and spread the fruits of digital technologies to more people in our region.

促进创新增长和数字经济发展。创新是推动世界发展的重要动力。我们要坚持创新驱动发展，把数字经济打造成增长新引擎，让数字技术成果惠及本地区更多的人民。

5. Countries need to seize the opportunities presented by the new round of technological and industrial revolution, strengthen cooperation in frontier sectors such as digital economy, artificial intelligence and nanotechnology, and work together to foster new technologies, new industries, and new forms and models of business.

各国应把握住新一轮科技革命和产业变革带来的机遇，加强数字经济、人工智能、纳米技术等前沿领域合作，共同培育新技术、新产业、新业态、新模式。

6. Guided by the conviction that "17 plus 1 could make more than 18", we have set up a multi-dimensional cooperation framework led by the leaders' summit and covering 20-plus sectors to ensure the participation of all CEE countries.

我们秉持"17+1 大于 18"的信念，建立了以领导人会晤机制为引领，涵盖 20 多个领域的全方位合作架构，以确保中东欧国家都能参与。

Part IV Vocabulary Treasure

1. **solidarity** *n.* a union of interests or purposes or sympathies among members of a group

   These achievements show the power of determination and global **solidarity**, but they also remind us of the challenges.

   这些成就显示了决心和全球团结的力量，但它们也提醒我们关注挑战。

2. **participation** *n.* the act of sharing in the activities of a group

   Teachers often encourage class **participation**.

   课堂上教师经常鼓励学生积极参与。

3. **benefit** *n.* something that aids or promotes well-being

   He had the **benefit** of a good education.

   他受过良好的教育。

4. **frontier** *n.* an undeveloped field of study; a topic inviting research and development

   The move is part of China's broader push to widen the application of

5G plus industrial internet, a **frontier** widely seen by countries around the world as key to boosting manufacturing prowess.

此举是中国扩大 5G＋工业互联网应用的更广泛努力的一部分，世界各国普遍认为这一前沿领域是提升制造业实力的关键。

5. **comprehensive**   *adj.*   including all or everything; broad in scope

Located at a geographical backwater, Ningxia has wasted no time in catching up with the wave of development in the e-commerce industry by setting up a **comprehensive** cross-border e-commerce pilot zone.

宁夏地处内陆，却不失时机地在电商产业发展的浪潮中奋起直追，设立了跨境电商综合试验区。

6. **inclusive**   *adj.*   including much or everything; and especially including stated limits

The digital economy is **inclusive**, social and flexible. People with disabilities can start their own businesses online, and many counties in China have traded their agricultural products online and become better off.

数字经济具有包容性、社会性和灵活性。残疾人可以在网上创业，中国的许多县已经实现了农产品网上交易，变得更加富裕。

7. **reap**   *v.*   gather, as of natural products

The painting depicted a group of peasants **reaping** a harvest of fruits and vegetables.

这幅画描绘了一群农民正在收获水果和蔬菜的情景。

8. **propel**   *v.*   cause to move forward with force; give an incentive for action

The tiny rocket is designed to **propel** the spacecraft toward Mars.

微型火箭的设计目的是推动太空船前往火星。

Part V   Language Practice

1. Translate the following paragraph into Chinese.

Humanity has created a colorful global civilization in the long course of its development, and the civilization of China is an important component of the world civilization harboring great diversity. As a representative feature of Chinese civilization, traditional Chinese medicine (TCM) is a medical science that was formed and developed in the daily life of the people and in the process of their fight against diseases over thousands of years. It has made a great contribution to the nation's procreation and the country's prosperity, in addition to producing a positive impact on the progress of human civilization.

2. Critical Thinking

This part is to improve the critical thinking ability by writing a composition.

Direction: Write a composition on the topic: Why do science and technology change our life? The composition is based on the following information, and it is at least 120 words.

 ➢ **the advancement of science and technology**
 ➢ **innovation, creativity and convenience**
 ➢ **my opinion**

Part VI   Further Reading

Chang'e-5, comprising an orbiter, a returner, a lander, and an ascender, with a total takeoff mass of 8.2 tons, is expected to accomplish unmanned rendezvous and docking in lunar orbit. After it enters the lunar orbit, the lander-ascender combination will separate from the orbiter-returner combination. While the orbiter-returner orbits about 200 km above the lunar surface, the lander-ascender will touch down on the northwest region of Oceanus Procellarum, also known as the Ocean of Storms, on the near side of the moon in early December.

About 2 kg of samples are expected to be collected and sealed in a container in the spacecraft. Then the ascender will take off with the sample, and dock with the orbiter-returner in orbit. After the samples are transferred to the returner, the ascender will separate from the orbiter-returner.

The combination of orbiter and returner will then depart the lunar orbit and return to the Earth's orbit, where the pair will break up and the returner will conduct a host of complicate maneuvers to return to a preset landing site in North China's Inner Mongolia autonomous region in mid-December. The entire mission is scheduled to last about 23 days, according to the China National Space Administration.

Project planners have allowed the lander-ascender combination to work about two days on the moon to accomplish its major tasks—using a drill to obtain underground samples from 2 meters beneath the surface and a mechanical arm to gather surface dirt.

Experts explained that planners needed to leave sufficient time for the craft to perform the sophisticated collection operations in case of possible malfunctions, adding that the completion ahead of schedule indicates related apparatus worked very well.

Before the drilling operation began, the lunar soil measurement instrument mounted on the lander surveyed and analyzed the subsurface structure of the drilling point to prepare for the drilling.

During the entire collection process, engineers synchronized a full-scale simulation on mock lunar soil inside a laboratory in Beijing based on data of the real landing site's environment sent back by the lander-ascender combination in an attempt to observe and support Chang'e 5's operations on the moon, according to the space administration.

The next step in this landmark mission will involve the ascender, which will use its 3,000-newton-thrust engine to lift itself to lunar orbit to rendezvous and dock with the reentry capsule. It will transfer the lunar samples to the module and then separate from it. Through the program, China has acquired the basic technologies of unmanned lunar exploration with limited investment. To pave the way for manned lunar exploration and deep space exploration, the Chang'e-5 mission will use a sampling method different to those of the United States and the former Soviet Union. The United States sent astronauts to the moon to collect samples. In the former Soviet Union's unmanned lunar sampling missions, the spacecraft took off from the moon and returned to the Earth directly. But China chose a complicated technological approach including unmanned rendezvous and docking in lunar orbit, which could bring back more samples and lay a technological foundation for manned lunar missions. At the same time, Chang'e 5 is also tasked with verifying key technologies such as lunar takeoff, lunar orbital rendezvous and docking and lunar sample storage, to accumulate important technology for China's future manned lunar landing and deep space exploration.

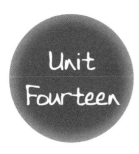

Unit Fourteen

Cultural Diversity

Part I Pre-Reading Task

Held every year on 21 May, the World Day for Cultural Diversity for Dialogue and Development celebrates not only the richness of the world's cultures, but also the essential role of intercultural dialogue for achieving peace and sustainable development. The United Nations General Assembly first declared this World Day in 2002, following UNESCO's adoption of the 2001 Universal Declaration on Cultural Diversity, recognizing the need to "enhance the potential of culture as a means of achieving prosperity, sustainable development and global peaceful coexistence."

The World Day for Cultural Diversity for Dialogue and Development is an occasion to promote culture and highlight the significance of its diversity as an agent of inclusion and positive change. It represents an opportunity to celebrate culture's manifold forms, from the tangible and intangible, to creative industries, to the diversity of cultural expressions, and to reflect on how these contribute to dialogue, mutual understanding, and the social, environmental and economic vectors of sustainable development.

All are invited to join in, and promote the values of cultural diversity, dialogue and development across our globe.

Questions:

1. Which day is the World Day for Cultural Diversity?

2. What does the World Day for Cultural Diversity represent?

3. Why do we need the World Day for Cultural Diversity?

Part II   Reading Task

- In the best Chinese tradition, they were *bazheshoujiao*—"teaching by holding his hand"—so much so that he would happily come back for more.

But assuming that the contrast I have developed is valid, and that the fostering of skills and creativity are both worthwhile goals, the important question becomes this: Can we gather, from the Chinese and American extremes, a superior way to approach education, perhaps striking a better balance between the poles of creativity and basic skills?

Questions:

1. What are the pros and cons of the Chinese way of teaching—"*bazheshoujiao*"?

2. How to strike a balance between the Chinese and American extremes of education?

3. Do you think that Chinese education and Western education can arrive at the same destination via different routes?

- **Valentine's Day**, also called **St. Valentine's Day**, is a holiday (February 14) when lovers express their affection with greetings and gifts. Given their similarities, it has been suggested that the holiday has origins in the Roman festival of Lupercalia, held in mid-February. The festival, which celebrated the coming of spring, included fertility rites and the pairing off of women with men by lottery. At the end of the 5th century, Pope Gelasius I forbid the celebration of

Lupercalia and is sometimes attributed with replacing it with St. Valentine's Day, but the true origin of the holiday is vague at best. Valentine's Day did not come to be celebrated as a day of romance until about the 14th century. Valentine's Day is celebrated on Sunday, February 14, 2021.

Qixi Festival, also called the Double Seventh Festival, on the seventh day of the seventh lunar month, is a traditional festival full of romance.

This festival is in mid-summer when the weather is hot and the grass and trees show their luxurious green. At night, when the sky is dotted with stars, people can see the Milky Way spanning from the north to the south. On each bank of it there is a bright star which looks at each other from afar. One of the stars is thought to be the Weaver Maid and the other the Cowherd. There is a beautiful love story about them passing down from generation to generation.

Although today some traditional customs are still observed in rural areas of China, many have been weakened or diluted in cities. However, the legend of the Cowherd and Weaver Maid has taken root in the hearts of people. And the seventh day of the seventh lunar month has been regarded as China's Valentine's Day.

Questions:

1. What is the similarity between the stories behind Valentine's Day and Qixi Festival?
2. Do you know the romantic story of the Cowherd and the Weaver Maid? Please tell the story to your classmates.
3. Do you agree with the famous Chinese saying that "If love between both sides can last for aye, why need they stay together night and day"?

● Spaghetti was still a little known foreign dish in those days. Neither Doris nor I had ever eaten spaghetti, and none of the adults had enough experience to be good at it. All the good humor of Uncle Allen's house reawoke in my mind as I recalled the laughing arguments we had that night about the socially respectable method for moving spaghetti from plate to mouth.

"Now, boys," he said. "I want to read you an essay. This is titled, 'The Art of Eating Spaghetti.'"

Questions:

1. What is the decent way to eat spaghetti?
2. Why does the author say that eating spaghetti is an art?
3. Can you name three types of representative Chinese noodles?

• It's common to hear people say that the world is getting smaller, and that there are fewer differences between families in the East and in the West than there were even a generation ago. Some people also say that family life around the world is acquiring negative features associated with the West, and abandoning those positive ones associated with the East.

But some differences still remain, particularly in how the young and old are looked after within the family. The so-called nuclear family in the West comprises the immediate family of parents and the children living under the same roof. It is less common to include grandparents. It would be extremely unusual for a family to live with other members of the extended family, such as uncles and aunts.

Questions:

1. Which family members are usually included in a nuclear family in the West?
2. How are the young and the old looked after in a typical Chinese family?
3. What are the benefits of traditional Chinese family structure?

• In ancient China, four well-developed areas in natural science were astronomy, arithmetic, agronomy and traditional Chinese medicine (TCM). In modern China, TCM is the only subject among those four that hasn't been surpassed by Western science, and it still plays a significant role in most Chinese people's life. TCM is different from modern medicine in means of diagnosis, treatment, composition of drugs, and prescriptions.

Questions:

1. What are the four well-developed areas in natural science in ancient China?

2. What is the only subject among those four that hasn't been surpassed by Western science?

3. In what ways is TCM different from modern medicine?

Part III   Moral Tips

1. All people under heaven have the same goal, though they take different routes; they cherish the same concern, but they hold different views.

天下同归而殊途，一致而百虑。

——《周易》

2. If love between both sides can last for aye, why need they stay together night and day?

两情若是久长时，又岂在朝朝暮暮。

——秦观

3. Food security is among a country's most fundamental interests. Of all things, eating matters most, and food is the most basic necessity of the people.

粮食安全是"国之大者"。悠悠万事，吃饭为大。

4. There is no place more comfortable than men's own home no matter how simple and poor it is.

世界上没有一个地方比自己的家更舒适，无论那个家是多么简陋，多么寒素。

5. Good medicine is bitter in the mouth but good for the disease.
良药苦口利于病。

Part IV   Vocabulary Treasure

1. diversity   *n.*   the quality or fact of including a range of many people or things

Noting that **diversity** in human rights development should be respected, they expressed opposition to any attempt to politicize human rights and double standards, calling for a more equitable, just, and inclusive global governance architecture on human rights.

他们注意到应该尊重人权发展的多样性，表达了对任何将人权政治化和双重标准的反对，并呼吁一个更加公平、公正和全面的人权管理机制。

2. lunar   *adj.*   connected with the moon

Wang Chong maintained that solar and **lunar** eclipses, thunder, and rain were all natural phenomena, rather than signs of Heaven being displeased.

王充认为日食、月食、雷和雨都是自然现象，而不是上天不悦的表现。

3. vague   *adj.*   not clear in a person's mind

Preventing legitimate Chinese companies from US capital-market listings on **vague** national-security grounds only makes London, Hong Kong or Tokyo more attractive.

借模糊的国家安全理由阻止中国合法公司在美国资本市场上市，只会让伦敦、香港或东京更具吸引力。

4. spectrum   *n.*   *(usually single)*   a complete or wide range of related qualities, ideas, etc.

While the world ushers in a new era of multi-polarity, diversity of governance models across the ideological and cultural **spectrum** is anticipated and should be accepted with generous latitude for tolerance and inclusiveness.

在世界迎来多极化新时代的同时，意识形态和文化范围内治理模式的多样性是可以预见的，而且我们应该更加宽容和包容地来接受它。

5. **available**   *adj.*   (of thing) that can be used or obtained

In the past three years, Beijing has installed barrier-free facilities in 336,000 places, built 100 wheelchair-accessible streets and blocks, and established 100 "convenient life circles" with services **available** within 15 minutes of residents' homes, Beijing Daily reported.

据《北京日报》报道，近三年来，北京在33.6万个地方安装了无障碍设施，建成了100条无障碍街道和街区；建立了100个"便民生活圈"，提供15分钟内上门的服务。

6. **diagnosis**   *n.*   (of sth) the act of discovering or identifying the exact cause of an illness or a problem

This not only shows that the authorities' decision to support the development of internet-based medical **diagnosis** and treatment services has helped, but also that patients are increasingly trusting internet-based medical service providers.

这不仅表明当局支持互联网医疗诊疗服务发展的决定是正确的，而且表明患者越来越信任基于互联网所提供的医疗服务。

Part V   Language Practice

1. Translate the following sentences into English.

（1）文化上，坚持尊重世界文明多样性，以文明交流超越文明隔阂，文明互鉴超越文明冲突，文明共存超越文明优越。

（2）百花齐放、百家争鸣，应该成为我国发展科学，繁荣文学艺术的方针。

2. Translate the following paragraph into Chinese.

Human civilization has been diverse since the very beginning, and diversity embodies the essence of civilization. The UNESCO Convention on the Protection and Promotion of the Diversity of Cultural Expressions states that cultural diversity forms a common heritage of humanity and should be cherished and preserved for the benefit of all; that cultural diversity creates a rich and varied world, which increases the range of choices and nurtures human capacities and values, and therefore is a mainspring for sustainable development for communities, peoples, and nations.

3. Critical Thinking

This part is to improve the critical thinking ability by writing a composition.

Direction: Write a composition on the topic: My View on Cultural Diversity. The composition is based on the following information, and it is at least 120 words.

> ➤ **general introduction to cultural diversity**
> ➤ **the benefits and challenges of cultural diversity**
> ➤ **my opinion**

Part VI Further Reading

Cultural Diversity Leads to a Shared
Future for the World (excerpt)

All civilizations are of equal value, and all have merits and flaws. There is no such thing as a perfect civilization or a civilization without a single virtue, and no one civilization should be judged superior or inferior to another.

Before the opening of new sea routes, there existed a state of basic equality between different civilizations. This state was shattered, however, by Western colonial expansion and eventual hegemony. During this process, some remote civilizations were decimated, such as the American Indian and ancient West African civilizations, and core regions of ancient civilizations such as West Asia, North Africa, India, fell one by one into the hands of Western invaders. Equality between civilizations no longer existed, and many civilizations faced a crisis of life and death.

According to Arnold Toynbee, challenge and response constitute a mechanism for the existence of civilization that determines whether a civilization will disappear or continue. Whether this theory is correct or not, the fact is that at the moment of Western hegemony reaching its peak, at a time when many civilizations were facing a crisis of life and death, there formed a global movement, and that movement was named modernization. This marked the beginning of cultural rejuvenation, the means of which was modernization. Through modernization, non-Western countries learned from the West how to catch up. By the beginning of the 21st century, non-Western countries had already achieved tremendous progress toward modernization, ushering in a new historical turning point.

Modernization began in Western Europe, and the emergence of modern nation-states marked the starting point of this process, which involved all aspects of society. Many important events from the history textbook, such as the Renaissance, the Reformation, the opening of new sea routes, the scientific and technological revolution, and the bourgeoisie revolution, are all part of Western modernization. Today, while the process of modernization has generally been completed in Western countries, cultural diversity has not disappeared. On the contrary, it has become even more vibrant, even within those Western countries.

First, there are different pathways to modernization. Britain took a gradual approach toward reform, France took the road of violent revolution, Germany carried out reforms from the top down, and the US, as a British colony, had to first gain independence before focusing on development. On the economic front, after the Industrial Revolution, Britain adopted the laissez-faire approach, and France basically followed suit while making some alterations, while Germany took the extraordinary route of promoting rapid economic growth with state power. Although the US followed Britain's laissez-faire model, in the 20th century, it became the first developed capitalist country to carry out large-scale state intervention.

Second, different countries have different political and social systems. Politically, Britain practices constitutional monarchy, while the US adheres to the republican system. There are clear distinctions between the parliamentary and presidential systems, further widening the political gap between the two countries. Looking at electoral methods, Britain has adopted the "first past the post" system, while the US invented the Electoral College system. As for the "three branches of government," the US is the only developed capitalist country to have truly incorporated this into its institutional design, so the US system is hardly the typical model. In terms of social systems, European countries practice a welfare model, something that the US has refused to adopt, perceiving it as a hotbed for laziness.

Third, Western countries are not immutable throughout the development process. As examples of this, Britain shifted from a laissez-faire society to a welfare-based one, France cycled through revolution to reach reform, and the US abolished racial discrimination policies, acknowledging racial equality at least in legal terms. These changes prove that there are differing forms of modernization even within one country, and that cultural diversity is a normal state.

Does cultural diversity inevitably lead to conflict, and does conflict in turn lead to a life-and-death contest? In the eyes of the Chinese people, "the ocean is vast because it embraces all rivers." The modern world can accommodate a diversity of modern civilizations, and modernization will mold a richer and more varied world. After a century of effort to modernize, many old civilizations have gained new life, recovered their confidence, and rediscovered their identities. The inequality between civilizations caused by Western hegemony is now being reversed. In this complex and changing world, the only way to resolve humanity's common problems is to rely on the concerted efforts of all civilizations, both Western and non-Western ones.

Today's world has become a community with a shared future in which all countries are bound together. It is an irreversible trend of the times that people around the globe must join hands to overcome difficulties and achieve shared development. Everyone should uphold the idea of living in a rich, vibrant, and culturally diverse world, create a bright tapestry interwoven with elements of all civilizations, and work together to eliminate real cultural barriers, to resist erroneous views obstructing the interaction of human minds, and to eliminate misunderstandings hindering human exchange, and learn from one another in the modern world to create a better future for all.

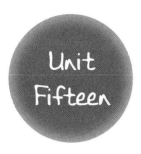

Unit Fifteen

Global Community

Part I Pre-Reading Task

"The ocean is vast because it admits all rivers." Openness and inclusiveness have made Geneva a center of multilateral diplomacy. We should advance democracy in international relations and reject dominance by just one or several countries. All countries should jointly shape the future of the world, write international rules, manage global affairs and ensure that development outcomes are shared by all.

In 1862, in his book *Un Souvenir de Solférino*, Henry Dunant pondered the question of whether it is possible to set up humanitarian organizations and conclude humanitarian conventions. The answer came one year later with the founding of the International Committee of the Red Cross. Over the past 150-plus years, the Red Cross has become a symbol and a banner. In the face of frequent humanitarian crises, we should champion the spirit of humanity, compassion and dedication and give love and hope to the innocent people caught in dire situations. We should uphold the basic principles of neutrality, impartiality and independence, refrain from politicizing humanitarian issues and ensure non-militarization of humanitarian assistance.

Questions:

1. Apart from the International Committee of Red Cross, do you know any other international health organizations?

2. What do you expect Chinese health workers to do in writing international rules and managing global affairs in the health field?

3. What kind of competencies should a Chinese health worker have if he or she wants to be involved in global health affairs?

Part II   Reading Task

• Although Einstein's five papers were published in a single year, he had been thinking about physics, deeply, since childhood. "Science was dinner-table conversation in Einstein household, " explains Galison. Albert's father Hermann and uncle Jakob ran a German company making such things as dynamos, arc lamps, light bulbs and telephones. This was high-tech at the turn of the century, "like a Silicon Valley company would be today," notes Galison.

Questions:

1. What do you know about the high-tech in the 20th century?

2. What do you know about high-tech in the 21st century?

3. Where is Silicon Valley? What's Silicon Valley famous for?

• Now, approaching another Thanksgiving, I have asked myself what will I wish for all who are reading this, for our nation, indeed for our whole world since, quoting a good and wise friend of mine, "In the end we are mightily and merely people, each with similar needs." First, I wish for us, of course, the simple common sense to achieve world peace, that being paramount for the very survival of our kind.

Questions:

1. Do you think we live in a peaceful world? If not, why?

2. Name a few places or regions where conflicts exist and wars might break out. Share with us the reasons why you think those regions are not peaceful?

3. What can China do to maintain a safe and peaceful environment for the very survival of our kind?

- WHO has identified six diseases whose worldwide re-emergence should be monitored: diphtheria, cholera, dengue fever, yellow fever, and believe it or not, bubonic plague. A list of diseases for the United States might differ, but, as Lederberg also put it, "We arrive at the realization that world health is indivisible, that we cannot satisfy our most parochial needs without attending to the health conditions of the globe." With a crowded marketplace in Kikwit, Zaire, site of the last Ebola flare-up, less than 24 hours away from a New York City subway, borders are meaningless to pathogenic microbes.

Questions:

1. What is emerging disease and what is re-emerging disease?

2. Do you think WHO's list of six re-emerging diseases are the same for every country in the world? If not, why?

3. In what countries do you think new diseases such as AIDS and Ebola have suddenly appeared and old afflictions such as TB, thought conquered, have flared?

- More and more people are in nursing homes at the end of life. In a nursing home, nursing staff is also always present. A nursing home, sometimes called a skilled nursing facility, has advantages and disadvantages for end-of-life care. Unlike a hospital, a doctor is not in the nursing home all the time. But, plans for end-of-life care can be arranged ahead of time, so that when the time comes, care can be provided as needed without first consulting a doctor.

Questions:

1. Ageing is a global problem. In your opinion, how do Western people and Eastern people treat their ageing population?

2. Why do many Western old people choose to go to nursing homes when they are old? How about Chinese people? What cultural differences can you learn from these differences?

3. Do you want to stay at a nursing home or at home when you are old? Why or why not?

● Identifying similar words, linguists have come up with what they call an Indo-European parent language, spoken until 3500 to 2000BC. These people had common words for *snow, bee* and *wolf* but no word for *sea*. So some scholars assume they lived somewhere in north-central Europe, where it was cold. Traveling east, some established the languages of India and Pakistan, and others drifted west toward the gentler climates of Europe. Some who made the earliest move westward became known as the Celts, whom Caesar's armies found in Britain.

Questions:

1. What languages do you think Indians and Pakistanis speak? Do you think their languages have something in common?

2. Besides Indo-European language family, there are other language families, such as Niger-Congo language families, and Afro-Asiatic language families. Which family do you think Chinese belongs to?

3. There are different language groups, like the Germanic group, the Celtic group, the Roman group and the Slavic group under Indo-European language families. In which groups do English, German, French, Spanish, Italian and Russian belong to respectively?

Part III   Moral Tips

1. Under framework of the Belt and Road Initiative, China-Africa cooperation has strengthened, with 52 African countries and the African Union Commission signing cooperation agreements with China. While many railway, road, airport, port and power station projects have been completed, many others are under construction or in the planning stage, which are expected to boost the socioeconomic development of Africa in general and the DR Congo in particular.

在"一带一路"倡议下，中非继续加强合作，52 个非洲国家和非洲联盟委员会和中国签订了合作协议。许多铁路、公路、机场、港口和发电站项目已经完成，还有许多别的项目正在建设中或在规划阶段。这些项目有望促进非洲，尤其是刚果民主共和国的社会经济发展。

2. Each year the International Day of Peace is observed around the world on 21 September. The UN General Assembly has declared this as a day devoted to strengthening the ideals of peace, through observing 24 hours of non-violence and cease-fire.

每年的 9 月 21 日，世界各地都举行国际和平日庆祝活动。联合国大会宣布设立的这一节日通过践行 24 小时无暴力和停火行动，致力于增强和平的理念。

3. To strengthen the technical and strategic collaboration, WHO and the ANRS | Emerging Infectious Diseases signed a memorandum of understanding aimed at improving the scientific and technical cooperation between the 2 institutions in the area of HIV, hepatitis and STIs in low- and middle-income countries (LMICs), notably in west and central African countries.

为了加强技术和战略合作，世界卫生组织和法国国家艾滋病研究署传染病处签订了谅解备忘录，旨在提高两个机构在中低收入国家，特别是西非和中非，在 HIV、肝炎和性传播疾病方面的科学和技术合作。

4. The second France-Chinese Carbon Neutrality Cooperation Submit was staged to mark the seventh anniversary of the signature of the Paris Agreement, an important international treaty reached among more than 190 parties of the United Nations to address the problem of climate change.

正值《巴黎协定》达成 7 周年之日，第二届法中碳中和合作峰会今日举办。《巴黎协定》是一项重要的国际协定，由联合国 190 多个缔约方共同签署达成，以应对气候变化问题。

5. Worldwide, life expectancy of older people continues to rise. By 2020, for the first time in history, the number of people aged 60 years and older will outnumber children younger than 5 years. By 2050, the world's population aged 60 years and older is expected to total 2 billion, up from 841 million today. Eighty per cent of these older people will be living in low-income and middle-income countries.

世界范围内，老年人的预期寿命持续增长。到 2020 年，60 岁以上的老年人数量在历史上首次超过 5 岁以下儿童人数。到 2050 年，全世界 60 岁以上老年人数有望从今天的 8.41 亿上升到 20 亿。这些老年人中的 80% 将生活在中低收入国家。

Part IV   Vocabulary Treasure

1. **UNICEF**   *abbr.*   United Nations International Children's Emergency Fund, an agency of the United Nations responsible for programs to aid education and the health of children and mothers in developing countries
The United Nations Children's Fund (**UNICEF**) works in 190 countries and territories to save children's lives, to defend their rights, and to help them fulfil their potential, from early childhood through adolescence.

联合国儿童基金会（UNICEF）在 190 个国家和地区开展工作，拯救儿童生命，维护儿童权利；从幼儿时期到青春期，帮助儿童实现发展潜力。

2. **parliament** *n.* the group of people who are elected to make and change the laws of a country

The Houses of **Parliament** in Britain is divided into the House of Commons and the House of Lords. It's the legislature of the United Kingdom.

英国的议会分为下院和上院。它是英国的立法机关。

3. **navigation** *n.* the skill or the process of planning a route for a ship or other vehicle and taking it there

The 4 major global **navigation** satellite systems are GPS of America, BDS of China, GLONASS of Russia and GALILEO of EU. The Bei Dou Navigation Satellite System (BDS) has been independently constructed and operated by China.

全球的四大导航系统是美国的全球定位系统、中国的北斗卫星导航系统、俄罗斯的格洛纳斯和欧盟的伽利略系统。北斗卫星导航系统由中国自主建设运行。

4. **ethnic** *adj.* connected with or belonging to a nation, race or people that shares a cultural tradition

There are 56 **ethnic** groups in China, including Han, Tibetan, Uyghur, Mongolians, and etc.

在中国有 56 个民族，包括汉族、藏族、维吾尔族、蒙古族等。

5. **Mediterranean** *n.* a place connected with the Mediterranean sea or the countries and regions that surround it

The Suez Canal joins the **Mediterranean** and the Red Sea.

苏伊士运河连接着地中海和红海。

6. **statistics** *n.* a collection of information shown in numbers

UN **statistics** show that around 1 million animal and plant species are threatened with extinction more than ever before in human history.

联合国统计数字显示约有一百万个动植物种类有濒临灭绝的威胁，这比人类历史上任何时候都要多。

7. **resilience**   *n.*   the ability of people or things to feel better quickly after sth. unpleasant , such as shock, injury, etc.

By strengthening the **resilience** of industrial and supply chains, China has helped ease the inflation pressure globally.

通过增强工业和供应链的韧性，中国帮助缓解了全球的通胀压力。

Part VI   Language Practice

1. Translate the following paragraphs into English.

中国积极参与全球治理体系改革和建设，践行共商共建共享的全球治理观，坚持真正的多边主义，推进国际关系民主化，推动全球治理朝着更加公正合理的方向发展。坚定维护以联合国为核心的国际体系、以国际法为基础的国际秩序、以联合国宪章宗旨和原则为基础的国际关系基本准则，反对一切形式的单边主义，反对搞针对特定国家的阵营化和排他性小圈子。推动世界贸易组织、亚太经合组织等多边机制更好发挥作用，扩大金砖国家、上海合作组织等合作机制影响力，增强新兴市场国家和发展中国家在全球事务中的代表性和发言权。

中国坚持积极参与全球安全规则制定，加强国际安全合作，积极参与联合国维和行动，为维护世界和平和地区稳定发挥建设性作用。构建人类命运共同体是世界各国人民前途所在。万物并育而不相害，道并行而不相悖。只有各国行天下之大道，和睦相处、合作共赢，繁荣才能持久，安全才有保障。中国提出了全球发展倡议、全球安全倡议，愿同国际社会一道努力落实。中国坚持对话协商，推动建设一个持久和平的世界；坚持共建共享，推动建设一个普遍安全的世界；坚持合作共赢，推动建设一个共同繁荣的世界；坚持交流互鉴，推动建设一个开放包容的世界；坚持绿色低碳，推动建设一个清洁美丽的世界。

2. Critical Thinking

This part is to improve the critical thinking ability by writing a composition.

Direction: Write a composition on the topic: Should euthanasia (安乐死) be legalized? The composition is based on the following information, and it's at least 120 words.

> ➢ **legal in some countries**

> ➢ **illegal in most countries**

> ➢ **my opinion**

Part VI   Further Reading

Remarks by Chinese President Xi Jinping at the Global Health Summit (excerpt)

In this unprecedented battle against the pandemic, China has, while receiving support and help from many countries, mounted a massive global humanitarian operation. At the 73rd World Health Assembly held in May last year, I announced five measures that China would take to support global anti-pandemic cooperation. Implementation of those measures is well underway. Notwithstanding the limited production capacity and enormous demand at home, China has honored its commitment by providing free vaccines to more than 80 developing countries in urgent need and exporting vaccines to 43 countries. We have provided 2 billion US dollars in assistance for the COVID–19 response and economic and social recovery in developing countries hit by the pandemic. We have sent medical supplies to more than 150 countries and 13 international organizations, providing more than 280 billion masks, 3.4 billion protective suits and 4 billion testing kits to the world. A cooperation mechanism has been established for Chinese hospitals to pair up with 41 African hospitals, and construction for the China-assisted project of the Africa CDC headquarters officially started at the end of last year.

Important progress has also been made in the China-UN joint project to set up in China a global humanitarian response depot and hub. China is fully implementing the G20 Debt Service Suspension Initiative for Poorest Countries and has so far put off debt repayment exceeding 1.3 billion US dollars, the highest deferral amount among G20 members.

In continued support for global solidarity against COVID-19, I wish to announce the following:

— China will provide an additional 3 billion US dollars in international aid over the next three years to support COVID-19 response and economic and social recovery in other developing countries.

— Having already supplied 300 million doses of vaccines to the world, China will provide still more vaccines to the best of its ability.

— China supports its vaccine companies in transferring technologies to other developing countries and carrying out joint production with them.

— Having announced support for waiving intellectual property rights on COVID-19 vaccines, China also supports the World Trade Organization and other international institutions in making an early decision on this matter.

— China proposes setting up an international forum on vaccine cooperation for vaccine-developing and producing countries, companies and other stakeholders to explore ways of promoting fair and equitable distribution of vaccines around the world.

Colleagues,

The ancient Roman philosopher Seneca said, "We are all waves of the same sea." Let us join hands and stand shoulder to shoulder with each other to firmly advance international cooperation against COVID-19, build a global community of health for all, and work for a healthier and brighter future for humanity.